WHAT YOU ☜ SO-AZT-111 KNOW
ABOUT OVER-THE-COUNTER
MEDICATIONS CAN HURT YOU!

It's almost impossible to avoid the blizzard of non-prescription drug advertising—but you don't have to be snowed by it! Rely on *THE OVER-THE-COUNTER DRUG BOOK* for comprehensive, authoritative information on more than 3,000 over-the-counter medications.

An informed consumer is a safe consumer. Learn:

- How to avoid the common cold—and choose the best cold remedies, if you do have one
- Why some "antiaging" skin products can actually accelerate the aging process
- Which over-the-counter drug ingredients may cause abnormal sensitivity to sunlight
- How to find the information you need to know on a product label
- Which toothpaste ingredient is a highly effective cavity fighter—but must be used with caution by children
- Surprising information about mouthwashes that contain alcohol . . . and much more.

THE OVER-THE-COUNTER DRUG BOOK

Books by Michael B. Brodin, M.D.

The Encyclopedia of Medical Tests
The Over-the-Counter Drug Book

Published by POCKET BOOKS

THE OVER-THE-COUNTER DRUG BOOK

MICHAEL B. BRODIN, M.D.

POCKET BOOKS

New York   London   Toronto   Sydney   Tokyo   Singapore

The ideas, procedures, and suggestions in this book are not intended as a substitute for the medical advice of a trained health professional. All matters regarding your health require medical supervision. Consult your physician before adopting the suggestions in this book, as well as about any condition that may require diagnosis or medical attention. In addition, the statements made by the author regarding certain products and services represent the views of the author alone, and do not constitute a recommendation or endorsement of any product or service by the publisher. The author and publisher disclaim any liability arising directly or indirectly from the use of the book, or of any products mentioned herein.

An *Original* Publication of POCKET BOOKS

POCKET BOOKS, a division of Simon & Schuster Inc.
1230 Avenue of the Americas, New York, NY 10020

ISBN: 0-671-01380-7

First Pocket Books printing November 1998

10 9 8 7 6 5 4 3 2 1

POCKET and colophon are registered trademarks of Simon & Schuster Inc.

Cover photos by Tai Lam Wong

Printed in the U.S.A.

Notice

The purpose of this book is education. It is not intended as a substitute for the advice of a physician or as a handbook for self-diagnosis.

A desire to take medicine is, perhaps, the great feature which distinguishes man from other animals.

—Sir William Osler

Contents

○○○

SUBJECTS   1

Consultants

○○○

Andrew Cheng, M.D. (Ear, Nose, and Throat); Manhattan Eye, Ear & Throat Hospital; Saint Vincent's Hospital of New York.

Anthony Clemendor, M.D. (Gynecology); Beth Israel Medical Center; Lenox Hill Hospital.

Joseph Davis, M.D. (Urology); Cabrini Medical Center; New York University Medical Center.

Zoovia Hamid, M.D. (Internal Medicine); New Rochelle Hospital Medical Center.

Vicki Levine, M.D. (Dermatology); New York University Medical Center.

Oddvin Lokken, D.D.S. (Mouth and Teeth); New York University College of Dentistry.

David McConnell, M.D. (Allergy); The Presbyterian Hospital in the City of New York; St. Anthony Community Hospital; Arden Hill Hospital.

Robin B. McFee, D.O. (General Medicine); University Medical Center at Stony Brook.

Donald Morris, M.D. (Ophthalmology); The New York Eye and Ear Infirmary; Montefiore Medical Center.

Michael Ruoff, M.D. (Gastroenterology); New York University Medical Center; Bellevue Hospital Center.

David Sibulkin, M.D. (Dermatology); St. Luke's-Roosevelt Hospital Center; The Presbyterian Hospital in the City of New York.

Consultants

Introduction

○○○

The inspiration for this book came from personal experience. I had a cold—otherwise known as an upper-
respiratory infection—and wanted some relief. In the drugstore I found the proper aisle soon enough, but was then
presented with quite a dilemma: the number of Cough &
Cold choices astonished and confused me. I was bewildered
by all the DMs, CFs, PEs, SFs, ESs, DXs, EXs, PHs, AMs,
and PMs. I wasn't sure whether I should buy a combination
product or individual ingredients, brand name or generic. I
didn't know if I should buy a little or a lot.

I now had two problems: I was sick *and* confused. And
I'm a doctor myself.

After getting over my illness I started to do a little
research and was almost immediately consoled, because I
discovered that almost everyone is confused, including
doctors, pharmacists, and the Food and Drug Administration (FDA) itself, not only by cough, cold, and allergy
products, but by analgesics, antacids, moisturizers, and
sunscreens, to name a few.

Buying an over-the-counter (OTC) product is hard for
three reasons:

- You have to diagnose yourself correctly.
- You have to decide whether you need treatment.
- You have to decide what that treatment will be.

When you treat yourself, you're often skipping an important part of the process of making an informed decision,
since the only things you have to go by are your own
symptoms. A symptom is not a disease, but an indication of
something else going on. Sometimes the symptom and the
diagnosis go hand in hand—acne is a common diagnosis in
a teenager with pimples—but sometimes diagnosis is diffi-

cult and potentially hazardous, as it would be to diagnose appendicitis in someone with vague abdominal discomfort, loss of appetite, and constipation.

Assuming that you do make the right diagnosis, you then have to decide whether or not you need treatment at all. Unlike your car or washing machine, the human organism contains the mechanisms for its own repair. You have to go to the mechanic when your car won't start, but you don't necessarily have to take a laxative when your bowels won't start. When you cut yourself, the first-aid ointment does not heal the wound; when you have a cold, it's not the decongestant that finally rids the virus from your body. All living things, right down to one-celled creatures, have their very own repair processes, as does DNA itself.

Finally, if you've gotten through the first two steps, you have to decide what the treatment should be, the right dosage, and how long you should take it. If you consider different strengths, package sizes, and forms (tablets, caplets, capsules, gelcaps, and liquids), it has been estimated that there are 300,000 distinct OTC products out there.

I hope this book will help to make your decisions easier. If it doesn't and you're still confused, nothing beats going to a good doctor.

How to Use This Book

○○○

This book is divided into three main sections: Subjects, Ingredients, and Index. Each is designed to fulfill a specific need.

Subjects

If you are sick or have a recurrent medical condition and want to know what's available over the counter (OTC) to treat it, try to find the appropriate chapter in the Subjects section. This can also be thought of as a symptoms section. The topics are arranged alphabetically. There will be a general discussion of the medical problems, conditions, or diseases in question, along with specific references to OTC and prescription medications. The text here includes **bold faced** references to active ingredients, details of which can be found in the Ingredients section.

Sometimes actual product names are discussed, but more often only the ingredient is mentioned. The reason for this is that the Food and Drug Administration (FDA) does not approve actual products themselves, but only their ingredients. Tylenol, for example, is the best known example of the the active drug **acetaminophen**, but there are numerous sources of OTC **acetaminophen** besides Tylenol. The same is true of **guaifenesin** and Robitussin. Unfortunately, the chemical names are often much longer, more difficult to pronounce, and harder to remember than the brand names, but that's the way it is. Manufacturers know this well and spend millions to find the catchiest names. Furthermore, it is important to know these ingredient names: there is no law that says that Tylenol must contain **acetaminophen** or that Robitussin must contain **guaifenesin**. They could both be reformulated tomorrow and you wouldn't know the difference unless you read the label.

At times a representative example of a brand has been included next to its chemical name, for example: **ibuprofen** (Advil). This is not to endorse the product nor to imply that the product is a superior form of the drug, but only to help the reader identify and remember the ingredient.

Ingredients

You will usually be referred to this section from the Subjects section but you might come here directly if you have read the label on an OTC product and you want to know more about an active ingredient. It should be noted that these are *active* ingredients only. Most products contain a number of other things such as vehicles and preservatives that have little to do with the actual effect of a product. Active ingredients are arranged alphabetically and follow this format:

Use

General class of the drug, what it is used for, and, sometimes, how it works.

Where found

Products in which the ingredient is found. Because of the constraints of space and the nature of certain chemicals, these lists will vary a good deal. Sometimes the ingredient is the only active one, but many times it is found in combination with others. Including all of these would require a book in itself, so this list will often be incomplete. It should be remembered that compositions of brand name drugs can change. Remember to read the labels and double check.

Recommended Dosage

The dose ranges and durations given here are generally those that have been approved by the FDA for self-medication. If your doctor recommends a different dose or duration, of course, follow his or her recommendation.

Adults are usually defined as anyone twelve years or over; when this is not the case, it is specified.

When appropriate, you will also find information here regarding food intake, safety for pregnant or nursing women, and drug interactions.

Side effects and overdosage

Unintended or adverse effects are listed here. Remember that if you take medications in larger amounts or for longer times than recommended you increase the chance of undesired effects.

Synonyms
Included here are not only other names for the ingredient but also ingredients that may be included under the general term.

Index
Included here are brand names, ingredients, and general topics. It does not list every brand name in existence. It is not meant to be exhaustive but, rather, representative.

SUBJECTS

○○○

SUBJECTS

o o o

1

ALLERGIES

What exactly is an allergy?

Although a complete explanation of allergies would require a complete explanation of the immune system itself, something that is outside the scope of this book, a simple way to think of an allergic reaction is as something your body does to get rid of a substance that is foreign to it and that it perceives as harmful.

For example, the swelling that commonly occurs in poison ivy is an attempt to dilute and weaken the offending substance with body fluids. The itching is an attempt to get you to scratch the stuff off your skin. The redness is an attempt to increase the blood flow so as bring more of the body's defenses to fight off the chemical invader, and so forth.

Allergies are good when they recognize and get rid of things like germs, but they are more of a nuisance when they launch an all-out attack on something as innocuous as grass pollen.

Although there are many different kinds of allergies, when someone talks about being allergic what he usually means is that he gets a runny, congested, and itchy nose and tearing, puffy, and itchy eyes at various times during the year. We'll call these symptoms *hay fever.*

Hay fever symptoms may appear like clockwork every spring, summer, or winter, but at times they are more erratic. In all cases, however, the essential problem is caused by inhaling particles in the air. Most often these particles include pollens, molds, and house dust. You may be allergic to any or all these things to different degrees. Hay fever is not triggered by foods. Pollens and molds create allergy *seasons,* whereas house dust is a constant *(perennial)* problem. Seasonal hay fever tends to be more severe than the perennial variety.

The symptoms are similar to those of a common cold, and it can be hard to distinguish between the two, although certain medical tests can help. See Table 4 in Chapter 6 for distinguishing features. Individuals with hay fever may also suffer from hives, asthma, and eczema.

Allergy testing to find out what inhalants are responsible is controversial. If you do have testing, either with skin or blood tests, you will probably be presented with a large sheet of paper listing the various substances to which you are allergic, such *Alternaria* or *Cladosporium* molds, or ragweed, tree, and grass pollens. It is also possible to be allergic to pets, cigarette smoke, and a host of other substances. Once you know the substances the problem is what to do about them. There are two choices, avoidance or desensitization.

Avoidance sounds fine in theory, but unless you live in a bubble, you will find it very difficult. Desensitization (allergy shots) does work, especially with pollens, but it is time consuming and expensive. That's why people most often take pills or tough it out.

There are four classes of OTC medications that are used to treat the symptoms that go along with hay fever type allergies. Strictly speaking, you should choose the product based upon the symptoms you are having, as detailed in Table 1.

Table 1. Treatment of hay fever symptoms

Symptom	Antihistamine		Cromolyn	Decongestant		Analgesic
	Internal	Topical		Internal	Topical	
itchy and watery eyes	X	X				
red and puffy eyes				X	X	
itchy, runny nose and postnasal drip	X		X			
stuffy nose			X	X	X	
headache and sinus pain				X	X	X

As you can see, technically speaking, a stuffy (congested) nose is different from a runny, itchy nose. This is because of the way the body chemicals involved in the allergic reaction work.

Although there are many combination allergy relief products, it is generally better to treat your symptoms with separate medications. You will understand their effects better and will have more control over them. If you find a combination of drugs that works particularly well, you might then select a product with the same ingredients for ease of use.

Antihistamines

The mainstay of treatments for hay fever and allergic symptoms in general is the large and useful group of drugs called antihistamines. To understand how they work it is good to understand a little about the powerful chemical called histamine.

Histamine is found in many animals and plants and has a number of effects on the body, such as widening (dilating) blood vessels; allowing blood vessels to leak fluid; stimulating the nerves that cause itching; and constricting the bronchial tubes in the lungs. Histamine also promotes the formation of stomach acid by stimulating what are termed $histamine_2$ receptors in the stomach lining (as opposed to $histamine_1$ receptors in allergies).

Antihistamines are drugs that block the effects of histamine. It is important to understand that they *block* histamine rather than decrease the production of it. This means that if the histamine has already been produced and has already started to make your nose itch, it is too late for the antihistamine to work. You have to have it in your system before the allergic reaction takes place. This is why a regular, steady dose of medicine is the best way to take any antihistamine. Take it to *prevent* symptoms, not to treat them. If you play catch-up, you're losing the game.

Histamine is responsible for roughly half of the symptoms of hay fever allergies; thus, you can expect about a fifty-percent reduction in your symptoms.

The following are the currently approved and available OTC antihistamines for allergy relief:

- **Brompheniramine**
- **Chlorpheniramine**
- **Clemastine**
- **Dexbrompheniramine**
- **Diphenhydramine**
- **Doxylamine**
- **Phenindamine**
- **Pheniramine**
- **Pyrilamine**
- **Triprolidine**

As a group, antihistamines are among the most widely used and versatile in medicine and they constitute a good portion of the OTC market in all categories. They are used not only for allergy relief but also to aid sleep, suppress coughs, and prevent motion sickness. In topical form they act as anesthetics. They also tend to be safe when used as directed. There are more antihistamines than those listed above and new ones are constantly hitting the market, most of them having been designed to reduce side effects.

For the most part, the most troublesome of these side effects is drowsiness, and much research has gone into finding non-sedating antihistamines. At present these are available only by prescription and include drugs such as Allegra (fexofenadine), Hismanal (astemizole), and Claritin (loratadine). All, however, are much more expensive and have additional drug interaction problems. By the way, there is no benefit to going to the doctor for a shot of antihistamine; the oral forms are actually preferable.

Although all OTC antihistamines carry the drowsiness warning, **brompheniramine, chlorpheniramine, dexbrompheniramine,** and **pheniramine** are the least sedating, whereas **clemastine, diphenhydramine,** and **doxylamine** are the most sedating.

One way around the drowsiness issue, but only for allergic eye symptoms, is to use antihistamines by way of eye drops. There are two OTC topical eye antihistamines, **pheniramine** and **antazoline,** which are similar but not exactly the same. Both are combined with the decongestant **naphazoline** for added effectiveness.

The drowsiness from antihistamines can be felt as weakness or fatigue and the effect is considerably worsened by alcohol or other sedatives. It's rather easy to forget this if you happen to be at a party, and you have to be very careful when driving. Sometimes, however, particularly in children or the elderly, antihistamines produce an odd and exactly opposite effect—agitation and insomnia. If this occurs there is nothing to do but discontinue the medication.

Other possible side effects include excessively dry mouth and nose, blurry vision, difficulty urinating, upset stomach, palpitations (rapid or irregular heartbeat), itching, rash, abnormal sensitivity to sunlight (photosensitivity), sweating, chills, thickening of lung secretions, and wheezing.

Antihistamines should not be taken if you have glaucoma, heart disease, thyroid disease, an enlarged prostate, diabetes, or high blood pressure. They should also not be taken with other sleeping pills, tranquilizers, or antidepressants such as monoamine oxidase inhibitors (MAOIs). You should check with your doctor if you have a lung disease such as asthma, emphysema, or chronic bronchitis,

Remember that, although antihistamines will dry out your nose, they will not unplug it. For that you need a decongestant.

Decongestants

Decongestants do not directly interfere with histamine or the allergic reaction but work indirectly: whereas histamine widens blood vessels, decongestants narrow or constrict them. When the blood vessels narrow, circulation decreases and with it the leakage of fluid that causes swelling of the mucous membranes.

Table 2 lists available decongestants and how they can be taken.

7

Table 2. Decongestants

	Oral	Nose (inhaler)	Nose (liquids)	Eye
ephedrine			X	
desoxyephedrine		X		
naphazoline			X	X
oxymetazoline			X	X
phenylephrine	X		X	X
phenylpropanolamine	X			
propylhexedrine		X		
pseudoephedrine	X			
tetrahydrozoline				X
xylometazoline			X	

Of the oral decongestants, the oldest and by far the most popular is **pseudoephedrine,** the best known brand name of which is Sudafed. It can be obtained both by itself and in many combination products. **Phenylephrine** and **phenylpropanolamine,** the other available internal decongestants, are almost always found in combination with antihistamines, analgesics, cough suppressants, and mucus liquefiers. Like the topical products, they work by constricting blood vessels, but they are also stimulants that are related to **epinephrine** (adrenaline) and so may produce nervousness, tremors, irritability, restlessness, and insomnia. They can also raise blood pressure and cause a rapid or irregular heartbeat. It is interesting to note that **phenylpropanolamine** is the only FDA-approved OTC appetite suppressant on the market.

Although short acting, decongestants work well and will help you to breathe better. The stimulant effect also has a tendency to produce a feeling of euphoria, which some people find beneficial when they become depressed by a long allergy season.

To avoid taking an oral decongestant you might want to consider a topical nasal preparation. The four available nasal spray and drop decongestants can be broken down as follows:

- Short acting (up to six hours of relief): **naphazoline** and **phenylephrine.**
- Intermediate acting (up to ten hours of relief): **xylometazoline.**
- Long acting (over ten hours of relief): **oxymetazoline.** These are usually marketed as 12-hour preparations.

Although these products are generally well tolerated over the short term, very fast acting, and free of systemic side effects, they have a number of significant disadvantages, including irritation of the nose and a condition called rebound congestion, in which the initial constriction in the blood vessels actually reverses itself after a few days of use. The symptom then becomes persistant nasal stuffiness despite ever-increasing doses of medication. This problem is more common with the short acting ingredients than with the longer acting ones. If you experience this side effect, the recommended treatment is to wean yourself gradually off the product while switching to a non-medicated nose drop or spray with plain **saline.** These are usually marketed as saline mists. If breathing is still a problem, try a systemic decongestant.

The other way to deliver decongestants locally to the nose is to use a nasal inhaler such as Benzedrex, which contains **propylhexedrine,** or Vicks Vapor Inhaler, which contains **desoxyephedrine.** Nasal inhalers lose their potency quickly and don't last long before reaching their expiration dates. They also tend to cake easily with dried mucus.

Of the four decongestants found in eye drops, **naphazoline** is probably the best tolerated. You can find out more about eye preparations in Chapter 12 (Eye Problems).

Sinus pain or headache

The sinus pain from hay fever is typically over your forehead and cheekbones. If the pain is severe, associated with fever, chills, or tenderness over the areas when you press or if it is accompanied by a thick greenish or greenish-yellow nasal discharge, you should definitely see a doctor, as you should if you have significant ear pain, since you may

9

have a bacterial sinus or ear infection that should be treated with antibiotics, drainage, or both. Some individuals have cup-shaped sinus cavities that do not drain well and in these cases surgery may be helpful.

In general, decongestants, either oral or nasal, are more specific for relieving sinus pain than analgesics, which only mask the problem. Still, taking one of the internal pain relievers, such as **aspirin, acetaminophen, ibuprofen, ketoprofen,** or **naproxen,** may provide relief.

Cromolyn

The FDA has recently approved a new drug that works differently from the usual medications used to treat allergies. It is called **cromolyn** and is available as a nasal spray under the brand name Nasalcrom. Unlike antihistamines, which compete with already released histamine for receptor sites on cells, **cromolyn** prevents the release of histamine in the first place. It is most useful when used prophylactically starting a week or two before the allergy season and continuing throughout it. At the present time it costs more than traditional methods of treatment, but the price should come down in the future. Unlike other nasal sprays, it can be used over a long time without developing rebound, and it is certainly worth a try if you don't like the side effects of the allergy medications you are taking now. Unfortunately, it does nothing for eye symptoms.

Recommendations

Try to discover what is triggering your symptoms. If they occur throughout the year, try to reduce house dust. If they occur when you're around your cat, avoid your cat. If they occur when you mow the lawn, don't mow the lawn yourself.

For daytime use, try one of the less sedating antihistamines, such as **chlorpheniramine** (Chlor-Trimeton) or **brompheniramine** (Dimetapp).

For nighttime use, try one of the more sedating antihistamines, such as **diphenhydramine** (Benadryl).

If nasal congestion—as opposed to sneezing, runny nose, postnasal drip, and itching—is dominant, then one of the systemic decongestants, such as **pseudoephedrine** (Sudafed) should be taken. With the exception of **cromolyn,** nose drops or nasal inhalers provide very short-term relief.

If you find yourself seriously debilitated by your symptoms, see a doctor. One of the nonsedating prescription antihistamines may be in order, or you may need consultation with an allergist for testing and desensitization.

should continue. With the occasional information given, a
drop or two of saline present in very show-group patient
lived. This showed similar distributed by their symptoms and demonstrated on the remaining production
self-important are being tried of within much 3 health
and with acclimatize factors are acclimation.

2

ALTERNATIVE MEDICINES

Alternative treatments, sometimes called complementary
medicine, come in and out of fashion, and there always
seems to be a new twist to an old theme. Among the most
popular recent additions is *Reiki,* in which a practitioner
adjusts the "energy flow" around a person's body without
actually touching the body. Many of these treatments
border on witchcraft, but they are quite popular, and a 1993
study in the *New England Journal of Medicine* showed that
about a third of Americans use such treatments at least once
a year. Interestingly, almost three quarters of these people
did not tell their doctors about it.

Although many treatments, such as acupuncture, acupressure, aromatherapy, Christian Science, moxibustion,
naprapathy, reflexology, homeopathy, and herbalism, can
be thought of as alternatives to scientific or Western medicine, it is only the last two that are be discussed here, since
they are the ones that provide products you can buy OTC in
many pharmacies and health food stores.

Homeopathy

The philosophy of homeopathy originated in the early
1800s with a German physician named Hahnemann, who
practiced by administering very tiny doses of substances
which, when given in larger amounts, produced the same
symptoms as the ones being treated. This system took off
like wildfire and Hahnemann became a millionaire at a time
when being a millionaire meant something. Homeopathy
has fallen in and out of favor over the years and is currently

undergoing a resurgence. One advantage to manufacturers and practitioners is that the products are very cheap to manufacture, since one drop of the active ingredient can provide doses for many thousands of people. These ingredients are sometimes diluted so much, in fact, that there are no molecules of them left, and one is left with nothing more than a mixture of water and alcohol. Homeopaths explain this by claiming that the water and alcohol "remember" the former presence of the drugs.

Nowadays, the remedies are frequently given a space to themselves in pharmacies and health food stores. They come in small bottles and are usually arranged neatly on the shelf and attractively labeled with the conditions for which they are indicated, such as arthritis, bedwetting, insomnia, incontinence, acne, headache, leg cramps, impotence, menstrual pain, constipation, fatigue, coughs, colds, or any other problem you can think of. The products are always labeled for symptoms, because homeopathic treatment, strictly speaking, does not aim to treat a disease itself but only its manifestations.

The good thing about homeopathic medications is that, if they are properly manufactured, they should be perfectly safe, since they are far too diluted to have any effects whatsoever on the body, much less any side effects. There are documented cases where children have ingested huge amounts with no detectable signs of illness. They work best if you are a true believer.

Possibly the most colorful homeopathic nostrum is for the symptom of lovesick melancholy. It contains the actual, bona fide tears—greatly diluted, of course—of a heartbroken young woman.

Herbs

Unlike homeopathic drugs, herbs and plant products often have profound effects on the body. Medical therapy, in fact, started with herbs thousands of years ago, and plants continue to be the source of many medications.

It's not hard to come up with examples: caffeine from the coffee bean, opium and heroin from poppies, nicotine from tobacco, and cocaine from the coca plant. Others are digitalis, which strengthens the muscular action of the heart and comes from the foxglove plant and marijuana, which is dried *Cannabis sativa.* The ingredient in many OTC external pain relievers, **methyl salicylate,** is actually oil from the wintergreen plant. **Thymol** comes from thyme, and **menthol** from peppermint. **Witch hazel,** an astringent which has been used for hundreds of years, is derived from the twigs of a shrub called *Hamamelis virginiana.* There are scores of others.

The question, therefore, is not whether a certain plant can affect your body but, rather, whether it is good for you to *allow* a certain plant to affect your body.

Because of the Dietary Supplement Health and Education Act of 1994, virtually any herb can be sold OTC as long as it is considered a nutritional supplement and as long as the seller doesn't make any health claims about it. The seller can make a statement about the effect of the substance on the body, but this statement must be followed by a disclaimer stating that the product, "is not intended to diagnose, treat, cure, or prevent" any disease. Since neither the manufacturer nor the FDA is able to give you information, you are left to rely on the often astounding claims made by clerks in health food stores, by alternative medicine literature, or on the Internet. There really is no source of good, sound, unbiased information about herbal medications. The only sure thing is that you can't believe anyone with a vested interest in the sale of the item in question.

Another big problem with herbs and plants is that little is known about the effects of their various constituents. Ginseng, touted to be good for one's sex life, cholesterol, blood, brain, liver, and thyroid, not to mention its anticancer and antiviral effects, contains dozens of separate chemicals whose composition and concentration are different depending on whether one is talking about Asian or American ginseng and on what year of its life it is harvested in (the fifth year seems to be best). Furthermore, some studies on herbs have been shown to be erroneous because they have used misidentified plants.

Some herbs, such as St. John's wort *(Hypericum perforatum),* have been the subject of intense study by reputable scientific journals, and in some parts of the world, most notably Germany, doctors prescribe it far more often than they do Prozac for depression. Some studies have shown that it does work better than placebo in moderate depression. The problem here is that very little is known about long-term side effects. Again, because of the lack of adequate oversight, many St. John's wort products found in health food stores are too diluted to have any effects. Many of them also contain a concoction of other plant extracts, such as kava root *(Piper methysticum)*.

Table 3 lists representative herbs and their main claims to fame. Some are available as extracts in pill, capsule, or liquid form, whereas others are designed to be brewed like tea.

Table 3. Alternative medicine botanicals

Substance	Indication
aloe vera gel	inflammation
bearberry	urinary infections
black cohosh	menstrual and menopausal symptoms
chamomile	intestinal disorders
chaste tree berry	menstrual symptoms
cranberry	urinary infections
echinacea	immune system problems
eleuthero	fatigue
ephedra (ma huang)	asthma
evening primrose	eczema
feverfew	migraine headaches
garlic	various
ginger	motion sickness and digestive disorders
gingko	impaired circulation to the brain
ginseng	fatigue and loss of sex drive
goldenrod	urinary infections
goldenseal	intestinal problems
grapeseed	antioxidant
hawthorn	heart disease
kava root	mood disorders
licorice	ulcers, coughs
melissa (lemon balm)	intestinal disorders, infections, herpes
milk thistle	liver disorders

Substance	Indication
pennyroyal	unwanted pregnancy
peppermint	intestinal disorders
pine bark	antioxidant
plantago seed	constipation
saw palmetto	prostate enlargement
slippery elm	sore throat
St. John's wort	depression
tea tree oil	antiseptic
valerian	insomnia and anxiety
willow bark	inflammation and pain

Some of these treatments are innocuous, such as rubbing the juice from a freshly cut **aloe** plant onto your skin or drinking cranberry juice or chamomile tea, but some are very dangerous, such as Ephedra, which contains **ephedrine** and **pseudoephedrine.** Its sale is banned in many states. Pennyroyal has been responsible for massive hemorrhage and coma in women who used it as a "natural" method of abortion. Kava root, whose ingredients affect the same parts of the brain as benzodiazepines (drugs related to Valium), has caused near coma in a man who took it with alprazolam (Xanax). There is a fairly high rate of allergic skin reactions to many herbs.

Recommendations

Never doubt or minimize the human capacity for self deception and the power of suggestion. In one study, red and blue placebo capsules were given to two groups of people, all of whom had been told that they were for sleep. The group receiving the blue pills swore they worked much better. When two other groups were given the same pills and were told they were stimulants, they said the red ones worked better.

Demand to see evidence. If it sounds too good to be true, it is. Remember that hucksters put down and make fun of science because science exposes fraud.

If you like natural treatments, stick with chicken soup (or vegetable soup if you're a vegetarian). If that doesn't work and you really want to try herbs, look for a controlled study in a university in which you will be monitored carefully. You'll still be a guinea pig, but you'll know more about what you're getting into. Perhaps it would be best to wait until adequate studies have been performed, the active ingredients in the herb in question purified, and the correct dose determined. You will then be in a much better position to judge whether the treatment is right for you.

3

ARTHRITIS

There are many different kinds of arthritis, each with varying degrees of severity ranging from mild to crippling. The major types are rheumatoid arthritis, osteoarthritis (degenerative or "wear and tear" arthritis), gout, infectious (septic) arthritis, and traumatic arthritis (due to injury). Virtually any joint can be affected by it and the types differ in outlook and treatment. Diagnosis is determined by physical examination, the pattern and location of pain, X rays, joint fluid analysis, and blood tests. Treatment, therefore, has to be individualized, and this is best done under medical supervision.

Trying to diagnose and treat your own arthritis can be dangerous. Of the two approaches to OTC relief, using external analgesics or internal analgesics, it is the latter that will most often be found useful. The trouble is that arthritis lasts longer than the ten days that the labels on internal OTC pain relievers say is safe. You then have to make a choice: live with the pain or defy the label. Taking lots of pain pills can lead to ulcers and intestinal hemorrhage, among other things. (Details on this can be found in Chapter 22 on pain).

In practice, however, the discomfort from arthritis, particularly osteoarthritis, the most common type, is intermittent and it is often not necessary to take pain medicine constantly. It also may be possible to anticipate trouble. If you know you will be walking, dancing, or exercising a bit more than usual, for instance, you might take some **acetaminophen** or other internal analgesic a few hours before the activity commences and be able to reduce both the pain and the amount of drug necessary to combat it. The use of glucosamine and chondroitin sulfate, sold as nutritional supplements, cannot be recommended at this time until more research has been performed.

Other types of arthritis, in particular rheumatoid arthritis, must be treated under a doctor's supervision, because the doses of medication usually far exceed the OTC limits. The treatment of gout, similarly, requires prescription medications.

4

ASTHMA

There really shouldn't be any OTC medications for asthma. First of all, since it is an impossible disease to diagnose yourself, you must be under medical supervision before any treatment is started. Second, if you are under a doctor's care, he or she will almost never recommend an OTC product. If you have asthma, never use any OTC asthma preparation unless your doctor tells you to, and always let your doctor know exactly what you're taking and how much.

Unfortunately, asthma is such a common problem and is becoming so much more prevalent that there is a certain degree of complacency about it. In places like the Bronx, New York, it has reached nearly epidemic proportions, and many schoolchildren carry around their inhalers as they carry around their books and pencils. Olympic athletes interviewed on TV blithley mention their asthma as if it were nothing more than a nuisance. Although there is a wide range of severity, asthma is potentially a very serious disease that can result in death.

Asthma is only one of many conditions that may cause wheezing, shortness of breath, or cough. Other lung diseases, such as chronic bronchitis, tuberculosis, fungal infections, sarcoidosis, lung cancer, emphysema, and blood clots in the lungs (pulmonary emboli), can cause similar symptoms. In addition, heart disease can and often does show up as shortness of breath.

Asthma is one of the atopic diseases, which include hay fever, eczema, hives, and allergies. It is also the most serious of these diseases because, whereas the swelling in eczema affects the skin and in hay fever the nose and eyes, in asthma it is the airway itself that swells and chokes off air flow.

The hallmark of asthma is wheezing—a whistling sound—as you exhale. Other symptoms may be shortness of breath, a feeling of tightness in the chest, and cough. Although asthma is typically chronic, meaning that it lasts for a long time, it is usually intermittent, occurring in the form of attacks that may last hours or days. It also varies greatly in severity.

One or more things can precipitate an attack, such as pollens, house dust, molds, or pets. A common cold, bronchitis, or the flu, tobacco smoke, exercise, or drugs such as aspirin may be the trigger. In some people emotional stress can bring on symptoms, although it is hard to say which comes first: someone in an acute asthmatic attack is often extremely apprehensive because of his inability to get enough oxygen.

The best treatment for asthma is almost always based on prescription medications—most often inhalers—not OTC products. The reason for this is that most treatment programs are based on reducing the inflammation that is at the heart of the problem, and the only way to do that is with prescription steroids—relatives of cortisone. There are no OTC steroid inhalers. The available remedies only help open up airways, they do not reduce inflammation.

One of the things your doctor will probably do is to classify your asthma by severity based on the frequency, duration, and severity of your attacks, along with the results of *pulmonary function testing*. The correct treatment is based on severity.

At present there are two OTC asthma products, **epinephrine**, which is delivered by inhaler, and **ephedrine**, which is available in pill form. The ingredients are related to one another. **Epinephrine** is also known as adrenaline, a hormone produced naturally in the adrenal gland. This is the hormone that produces a protective and stimulating effect if we are confronted by danger or something we perceive as dangerous. It increases the heart rate and blood pressure and makes us sharper mentally. It also opens up the bronchial tubes to help us breathe better. It is this last effect

21

that makes it and chemicals like it (called adrenergic) helpful in treating asthma.

Epinephrine inhalers are only indicated for the mildest symptoms in the mildest category of asthma, however.

In big, bold print the following warning is supposed to appear on all OTC inhalers: DO NOT CONTINUE TO USE THIS PRODUCT BUT SEEK MEDICAL ASSISTANCE IMMEDIATELY IF SYMPTOMS ARE NOT RELIEVED WITHIN 20 MINUTES OR BECOME WORSE. DO NOT USE THIS PRODUCT MORE FREQUENTLY OR IN HIGHER DOSES THAN RECOMMENDED UNLESS DIRECTED BY A PHYSICIAN.

If your doctor recommends one of these inhalers, follow the manufacturer's instructions with regard to proper use. Some solutions are designed for use with a rubber bulb. Side effects such as rapid or irregular hearbeat, increased blood pressure, tremor, and anxiety, are usually not seen if the products are used correctly, but may definitely be seen in overdoses.

Similarly, if your doctor has recommended OTC oral **ephedrine**—which is almost certainly *not* the case—follow his or her directions carefully for its use. At the present time **ephedrine** is the subject of some controversy since it is known to be used as a precursor for the illegal manufacture of amphetamines (speed). Pharmacies must keep accurate records of its sale, which is restricted in some states. It may very well be completely illegal by the time you read this.

Most oral asthma products containing **ephedrine** also contain **guaiafenesin** (Robitussin), which is used to liquefy mucus. Such drugs are called expectorants. Although well tolerated and generally safe, you should only use them if your doctor tells you to. The same holds true with any cough or cold remedy you might be considering.

A word about antihistamines. For many years, doctors discouraged their use in asthma, but thinking has changed, and it may be that your own doctor has recommended one, particularly if you also suffer from hay fever and the hay fever symptoms appear to be aggravating your asthma. You should not under any circumstances take antihistamines, or any other products designed to relieve asthma, on your own without talking to your doctor first. If indicated, one of the

OTC antihistamines discussed in Chapter 1 on allergies may prove useful.

Although OTC asthma drugs are almost worthless, there is an OTC asthma device, called a peak flow meter, which is extremely valuable, especially for those with the worst symptoms. These home devices measure your ability to move air out of your lungs and are accurate and early predictors of trouble. Two brands are available, Assess and Mini-Wright. Each comes in a standard and low range, the latter being for more severe cases. Your doctor can advise you on their proper use. Using a peak flow meter will greatly improve the control of your asthma.

Recommendations

Most asthma specialists find no place for OTC asthma drugs, and you shouldn't either. Prescription medications are far more effective and safer.

If you have bad asthma, however, the peak flow meter is indispensable.

5

CHOLESTEROL

Cholesterol is not the totally toxic substance many think it to be. In fact, it is present throughout the body, forming a valuable foundation for the synthesis of many hormones, and without it we could not live. Its bad reputation stems from the link between high blood levels of it and coronary artery disease. Other causes of heart disease include sedentary life style, smoking, obesity, diabetes, uncontrolled high blood pressure, or a family history or personal history of cardiovascular disease. It is important to realize that all of these factors can be modified except for family and personal history.

There are two OTC ways to approach high cholesterol: home testing and drugs. Neither of them, unfortunately, is very good.

Unlike the valuable home glucose testing kits for diabetes, home cholesterol kits are almost worthless. In the first place, they only tell you your *total* cholesterol level, not what type it is. Cholesterol is carried in the blood in several forms (called fractions), each of which has a different function. Each of these fractions can be measured independently in the laboratory. Basically, what you want is high levels of high-density cholesterol (HDL) and low levels of low-density cholesterol (LDL). HDL cholesterol is good cholesterol, LDL cholesterol is bad cholesterol. Home testing does not give you any information about this.

Furthermore, for an accurate cholesterol determination, before you are tested your diet should not have changed for three weeks, your body weight should be stable, you should fast for twelve hours, you should not have consumed **alcohol**

24

for three days, and you should not have taken **vitamin C** or **acetaminophen** for four hours. Under these circumstances, if your blood cholesterol level is above 200, you should see a doctor for further testing.

Of the available OTC drugs that have been used in the past to lower cholesterol—**psyllium, aluminum hydroxide, and niacin**—none can be recommended without medical supervision. Furthermore, they are not approved for this use by the FDA, and for good reason: the amounts that have to be used produce too many side effects. You may also see advertisements or read articles extolling the virtues of chelation therapy with such things as grapefruit pills for cholesterol. These should be ignored, since there is no scientific evidence that they work.

In any event, before using any drug to lower your cholesterol, OTC or prescription, you should first take steps to change your diet, lose weight, and establish a good exercise program. It has been shown that losing as few as ten pounds will drop your cholesterol level significantly. For help, see Chapter 29 on weight reduction.

25

6

COMMON COLD

The illness we commonly call a cold can be caused by any of several types of viruses, each of which produces slightly different symptoms. The medical term for this is an upper-respiratory infection (URI), implying that the site of the problem is somewhere between the nose and the lungs. This is to distinguish these diseases from lower-respiratory infections of the lungs (pneumonia). There is no evidence whatsoever that cold temperatures, drafts, or damp, wet environments are to blame for the common cold. These myths persist because of two facts. First, colds are more common in the winter because of a generally dryer atmosphere and more crowded conditions inside buildings, both of which foster the spread of infection. Second, your nose tends to run when you are outside on a cold winter day. This secretion of nasal liquids is a nerve reflex called vasomotor rhinitis, and does not signify a cold or the onset of a cold. It is now known that the way the common cold is spread is almost always through hand-to-hand contact: one person has a cold, rubs his nose, sneezes, or coughs into his hand, which deposits the virus there, and it is then spread through touching someone else's hand. Breathing infected droplets from the air is possible, but less common. It is for this reason that you can reduce the number of colds you have every year if you wash your hands regularly.

Cold symptoms closely mimic hay fever allergy symptoms and it is often difficult to tell them apart. In many ways it doesn't matter, since OTC remedies are designed for both anyway, but you're more likely to feel better if you diagnose things correctly. Distinguishing features are listed in Table 4.

Table 4. Hay fever and cold symptoms

	Hay fever	Common cold
symptoms (in addition to a runny, stuffy nose)	itching of eyes, nose, or roof of mouth; postnasal drip; red, swollen, and teary eyes	Aches, pains, sore throat, cough; children may have fever
time of year	pollen season or constantly throughout the year	usually winter
other features	asthma, eczema, hives, or allergies in self or family; worse around animals, smoke, or dust	none

Lots of people throw around the term flu as if it were the same as a cold. The flu, however, which is medically termed influenza, is a much more serious illness, with very high fever, extreme weakness, headache, and lots of discomfort. Influenza is often so bad that the young, the old, and the debilitated may die from it.

It is said that a cold will go away in a week with treatment, and seven days without treatment, and this is still more or less true, except that the duration can often be two weeks, with some lingering symptoms, such as morning congestion or a dry cough, lasting even longer. Each cold virus has its own peculiarities, but you are more likely to classify your illness as mild, moderate, or severe. More helpful from the standpoint of treatment with OTCs is to divide up your symptoms and treat each accordingly.

Try to avoid combination cough, cold, and allergy products. These usually contain a decongestant, such as **pseudoephedrine**, **phenylephrine**, or **phenylpropanolamine**, an antihistamine, such as **brompheniramine**, **chlorpheniramine**, **clemastine**, **dexbrompheniramine**, **diphenhydramine**, **doxylamine**, **phenindamine**, **pheniramine**, **pyrilamine**, or **triprolidine**, an analgesic, such as **acetaminophen**, **aspirin**, **sodium salicylate**, or **ibuprofen**, a cough suppressor (**dextromethorphan**), and a mucus liquefying agent (**guaiafenesin**). Although they may be less expensive and more convenient than buying separate ingredients, there are a number of advantages to taking the drugs separately.

First, not all symptoms of a cold come at the same time. You may start with aches and pains, then develop a sore throat, then go on to nasal congestion and sneezing, then to a cough. Each symptom needs a different drug.

Second, you can individualize the dose of an ingredient and do not have to take the amount in the combination.

Third, you can substitute a more effective or better tolerated ingredient instead of having to take the one supplied. You might decide you want to take **ibuprofen** (Advil), for example, instead of **acetaminophen** (Tylenol) for pain, or vice versa.

Fourth, you won't get into trouble by taking extra medication.

Fifth, you don't have to take the antihistamine that is in almost all combinations. Antihistamines have little role in the treatment of a cold except to help you to sleep at night. If that's the problem, you can take a proper dose of a sedating antihistamine for sleep.

Seventh, you have complete control over what you are taking. Vicks NyQuil, a very popular product, contains **pseudoephedrine, doxylamine, acetaminophen, dextromethorphan,** and **alcohol** (ten percent). Although the **alcohol** is listed as inactive, it can have a significant effect if you take too much. Furthermore, warning labels both for **doxylamine** and **acetaminophen** clearly warn against taking with **alcohol.**

Eighth, and last, combination products are confusing. There are too many ingredients in too many (over four hundred) products. Here are some examples from the Alka-Seltzer product line:

Alka-Seltzer Plus Cold & Cough Medicine Effervescent Tablets: **aspirin, chlorpheniramine, dextromethorphan,** and **phenylpropanolamine.**

Alka-Seltzer Plus Cold & Cough Medicine Liqui-Gels: **acetaminophen, chlorpheniramine, dextromethorphan,** and **pseudoephedrine.** (The same ingredients are found in Children's Tylenol Cold Plus Cough; Theraflu Flu, Cold & Cough Medicine, Original Formula; Theraflu Flu, Cold & Cough Medicine Maximum Strength Night Time; and Tylenol Cold Multi-Symptom Hot Medication.)

Alka-Seltzer Plus Cold Medicine Effervescent Tablets: **aspirin, chlorpheniramine,** and **phenylpropanolamine.**

Alka-Seltzer Plus Cold Medicine Liqui-Gels: **acetaminophen, chlorpheniramine,** and **pseudoephedrine.** (The same ingredients are found in Children's Tylenol Cold Multi-Symptom Liquid.)

Alka-Seltzer Plus Flu & Body Aches Formula Effervescent Tablets: **acetaminophen, chlorpheniramine, dextromethorphan,** and **phenylpropanolamine.**

Alka-Seltzer Plus Flu & Body Aches Medicine Liqui-Gels: **acetaminophen, dextromethorphan,** and **pseudoephedrine.** (The same ingredients are found in Sudafed Severe Cold Formula; Tylenol Non Drowsy Medication; and Tylenol Maximum Strength Flu Gelcaps.)

Alka-Seltzer Plus Night-Time Cold Medicine Effervescent Tablets: **aspirin, dextromethorphan, doxylamine,** and **phenylpropanolamine.**

Alka-Seltzer Plus Night-Time Cold Medicine Liqui-Gels: **acetaminophen, dextromethorphan, doxylamine,** and **pseudoephedrine.** (The same ingredients are found in Vicks Ny-Quil.)

Each symptom, therefore, should be treated individually. If you take the recommended amounts of each drug and follow a few basic rules you won't get into trouble combining remedies for cold symptoms on your own. These symptoms are:

- Sore throat
- Aches and pains
- Fever
- Stuffy, runny nose and sneezing
- Chest congestion
- Cough

Sore throat

A sore throat is most often due to a virus when it is part of the cold syndrome. Occasionally, and importantly, however, it may be caused by a bacteria, specifically the *Streptococcus* germ found in strep throat. This needs prompt medical attention, testing, and antibiotics. Features that are more typical for strep throat than for a cold include sudden onset of a very painful sore throat, severe aches and pains, and enlarged lymph nodes (glands) in the neck. The typical symptoms of a cold, in fact, are usually absent in strep throat.

Part of the discomfort of a sore throat from a cold can be alleviated by internal analgesics (see Chapter 22 on pain), but some relief can be obtained by local treatment with a lozenge or spray. Popular ingredients include **benzocaine, dyclonine, eucalyptol, menthol** (peppermint oil), and **phenol.**

Although these ingredients are classified as anesthetics, only **benzocaine, dyclonine,** and **phenol** really create an actual feeling of numbness when applied to the mucous membranes. The numbness doesn't last very long, though, and it is hard to get much relief if you follow directions, which usually advise against more than four doses or applications a day.

Lozenges or candies that contain **menthol** as their sole active ingredient, such as Cepacol, Fisherman's Friend, Halls, Luden's, Ricola, Robitussin, and Vicks, can be used more frequently. The strongest of these appears to be Halls Mentho-Lyptus Ice Blue Extra Strength Cough Suppressant Drops, each of which contains twelve milligrams of **menthol.** It is interesting that despite all of the advances of modern medicine, the comforting and refreshing sensation of peppermint remains the most popular remedy for our most annoying ailment.

Although some of these preparations may contain an antiseptic such as **hexylresorcinol, cetylpyridinium,** or **alcohol,** there is no good evidence that these help kill the germs that cause sore throats or assist the immune system in any way. They can safely be avoided.

Stuffy, runny nose and sneezing

The best medication for treating a stuffy nose is a decongestant, not an antihistamine.

Antihistamines, which do have a place in treating hay fever, are sometimes used in cough and cold remedies because they dry out mucous membranes, but this is only a side effect. You may remain just as stuffed up and may find it just as hard to breathe as before, although there is one study which found that **clemastine** provided some relief.

Most antihistamines are also effective sedatives and help with sleep.

The same decongestants that are used for hay fever allergies are used for colds, except that as a practical matter you don't need to consider them in eye drop form. Also as a practical matter, nasal inhalers are often undesirable because they soil so easily. The real choice is between using a systemic (oral) decongestant or a topical one in spray or drop form.

If you choose an oral decongestant and decide to take it by itself, **pseudoephedrine** (of which Sudafed is the best known brand name) is the drug of choice. Although the regular form is short acting and needs to be taken every four to six hours, longer-lasting, timed-release forms are available that give twelve or twenty-four hours of relief.

Although **pseudoephedrine** will work nicely to unplug your nose, it is also a stimulant. This is fine for the day when you're working or going to school but may prove troublesome if you're trying to go to sleep.

At night, therefore, you might try a smaller dose. A different approach is to mimic a nighttime cold aid like NyQuil by coupling a normal dose of decongestant with one of the more sedating antihistamines such as **doxylamine** (such as Nytol Maximum Strength). If you have a cough (see below), **diphenhydramine** would be a good choice. Although antihistamines will help you sleep, if you're really achy, don't forget an internal analgesic before bedtime. Sedatives don't do anything for pain and by themselves may even make it worse, leading to restlessness and nightmares.

Chest congestion

The feeling of tightness in one's chest is related to the feeling of tightness in one's nose and should be improved with decongestants. There is, however, another problem, which is the accumulation of mucus in the bronchial tubes (the tubes which lead from the trachea to the lungs). This can get to be quite thick.

Now, it is not at all certain that the feeling of tightness is related to the thickness of this mucus, but most people are familiar with the urge to cough the mucus up and spit it out.

This is the reasoning behind the use of mucus liquefying agents, called expectorants.

There is only one available OTC mucus liquefying agent currently approved by the FDA—**guaiafenesin** (Robitussin), but there is little scientific evidence that it helps. Still, since it is the only one available and since the side effects are minimal, it is a big seller. More important in loosening secretions is increasing humidity in the environment with a vaporizer or humidifier and making sure you take adequate fluids.

Cough

Before you decide on a cough suppressant, you have to decide whether your cough is a "good" cough or a "bad" cough. If you are coughing up mucus (sputum) and have what is known as a productive cough, you are getting rid of bad secretions, which is a good thing. Cough suppressants, therefore, are not recommended for productive coughs. If your cough is dry, on the other hand, and you're just hacking away, not coughing anything up, cough suppressant treatment is indicated, especially if the cough is interfering with sleep or work.

There are two ways to use cough suppressants, orally or by inhalation.

Orally, two or three drugs are available, depending on what state you live in. **Dextromethorphan** and **diphenhydramine** are approved everywhere, whereas **codeine** is not always available OTC.

Dextromethorphan is a derivative of morphine and is present in many cough and cold remedies alone or in combinations that are often denoted by the suffix DM. Unlike morphine, however, it has almost no pain killing properties and a low potential for addiction.

The antihistamine **diphenhydramine** (Benadryl) is also labelled for use as a cough suppressant but is probably less effective than **dextromethorphan**. Still, it is usually well tolerated and may be useful at night.

Menthol and **camphor** are available as inhalation (topical) cough suppressants. The best example is the time-honored Vicks VapoRub, a greasy concoction that contains both of these substances in addition to **eucalyptol** and a host of other aromatic ingredients such as cedarleaf oil, nutmeg oil, and **turpentine.** It is designed to be slathered on the throat and chest in a thick coat that is warmed and made volatile by your body heat, so that you breathe in the vapors, a type of aromatherapy invented before that term came into vogue. Although the manufacturer (Procter & Gamble) gives instructions for use in children over two, the American Academy of Pediatrics recommends against the use of **camphor** in children, so you should check with your pediatrician before using a **camphor** product (particularly one with a concentration over two and a half percent) on your child.

Although it can be scientifically shown that drugs can diminish the cough response somewhat, the evidence that they do so in the case of colds is not so good. As is true of mucus liquefiers, cough suppressants are generally safe and sell well. The role of belief and faith in the remedy also cannot be discounted. Breathing in peppermint (**menthol**) vapors gives most people a warm and cuddly feeling.

Aches and pains

The various muscle and joint discomforts (myalgias and arthralgias) can only be treated with analgesics. The safest remains **acetaminophen** (Tylenol), and it should be remembered that **aspirin** is best avoided in children and teenagers fifteen years of age and younger. For those who want something different, the NSAIDs **ibuprofen** (Advil, Motrin, and others), **ketoprofen** (Actron, Orudis KT), and **naproxen** (Aleve) can be substituted. For more information on these see Chapter 22 (Pain).

Fever

Fever with a cold is very uncommon in adults. If you do have a fever it is likely to be so low as not to need specific treatment. A high fever in adults is more usual with the flu. Children, however, more commonly have a moderate fever and may be given **acetaminophen,** but never **aspirin.** See also Chapter 13 on fever.

Recommendations

For nasal stuffiness, use a systemic decongestant. **Pseudoephedrine** (Sudafed and others) is the oldest and its side effects are less risky for people with high blood pressure than those of other products. You can take the recommended dose during the day. At night, if you have trouble sleeping, try a lower dose. If you can't use a systemic decongestant, try one of the long-acting nasal sprays with **oxymetazoline,** but not for longer than five days.

Candies, cough drops, and lozenges containing **menthol** help soothe sore throats and can help suppress a nonproductive cough.

For coughs, the mainstay of treatment is **dextromethorphan.** At night add **diphenhydramine.** It will also help you sleep.

For chest congestion, **guaiafenesin** is the only thing available. Although probably not too effective, it is safe. Drink fluids and use a humidifier.

For aches and pains, take **acetaminophen.** It will also help a sore throat.

7

CONSTIPATION

There is no clear definition of constipation, since bowel habits vary so widely. Different individuals have different expectations of how they want their bowels to perform and different sensations they describe as constipation. To some people it might be missing one day if you go every day or feeling bloated or experiencing stool that is too hard or firm. To others it might mean not being able to have a bowel movement at all unless they take a laxative. These symptoms, in turn, may be mild or severe and may occur occasionally or constantly.

In certain situations constipation is to be expected. As we age, for example, our bowels tend to become sluggish, just like the rest of us. Those suffering from certain neurological, endocrine, muscular, or intestinal diseases have decreased bowel movements, as do those who are bedridden from any cause or who have had certain types of surgery. Medications such as some analgesics, antacids, antidepressants, cholesterol lowering drugs, and antibiotics, may interfere with normal evacuation.

Although chronic constipation may be due to a variety of diseases, most often it is due to chronic neglect, habitually ignoring the urge to defecate until the mass of stool becomes dried out and compacted in the colon. If we were animals in the forest we would heed the call as soon as we felt it, which is by far the most healthy way to take care of one's intestines, but toilet training and social convention robs us of our spontaneity. Some people just carry it too far. This problem then can become progressive, the colon becoming ever more distended until the sensation of rectal fullness is lost. With this, the use of laxatives begins and becomes essential to bowel movements.

No matter how you define it and no matter what the cause of it and what you do to prevent it or help treat it, the fact remains that one's bowel movements are fundamental to one's sense of well being. One meaning of the word fundamental, in fact, means exactly that: pertaining to the part of the body upon which one sits.

Although this book is about drugs, if you're otherwise healthy but always constipated you ought to seriously consider some changes, particularly if you're sedentary or subsist on a diet without many fruits, vegetables, or grains. Bowels work best when stimulated. Changing behavior is not easy, because we are creatures of habit, but habits can also work for you if you take the time and effort and don't get discouraged. Exercising more and improving your diet will almost always help regularity and reduce your reliance on laxatives.

So, if you think you need a laxative, consider your diet and physical activity first. Also check on the possibility that a medication may be causing the problem. If that doesn't work, have a physical exam and routine lab work. You may have an intestinal problem or your thyroid may be underactive or you may be depressed. If everything checks out and your doctor recommends a laxative, your choices can be broken down into five OTC categories:

- Bulk producers
- Stimulants
- Hyperosmotics
- Lubricants
- Stool softeners

Bulk-producing laxatives absorb liquid and swell in the gut. The increased mass of stool then stimulates the muscles of contraction and evacuation. Examples are **malt soup extract** (Maltsupex), **methylcellulose** (Citrucel), **psyllium** (Metamucil), and **calcium polycarbophil** (FiberCon). In general, these are your best choices, because they are the safest and act most naturally. They usually work in twelve to twenty-four hours, but may take as long as three days. The only real caution is that each dose *must* be taken with adequate fluid, which means at least eight ounces of water, juice, soda, or other liquid. Otherwise, the substance may swell, block your esophagus (the tube that leads from your mouth to your stomach), and you may choke on it. The following warning, which should appear in bold print, is typically found on the labels for these laxatives: "Taking this product without adequate fluid may cause it to swell and block your throat or esophagus and may cause choking. Do not take this product if you have difficulty swallowing. If you experience chest pain, vomiting, or difficulty in swallowing or breathing after taking this product, seek medical attention."

Stimulant laxatives act directly on the muscles that contract the intestines. These products are very popular, and include **bisacodyl** (Correctol), **casanthranol, cascara sagrada,** and **senna** (Ex-Lax and Fletcher's Castoria). **Castor oil** is usually also considered a stimulant laxative, although it works slightly differently and considerably faster than the others. Stimulants should be taken on an empty stomach for fastest results. The best time to take them—except for **castor oil**—is at bedtime. This will usually produce a bowel movement the next morning. The main disadvantage of stimulants is that one may become too reliant on them.

Hyperosmotic (saline) laxatives, such as **magnesium hydroxide** (milk of magnesia), **magnesium sulfate** (Epsom salt), **magnesium citrate** (citrate of magnesia), and **sodium phosphate** (Fleet Phospho-Soda) suck water into the intestinal cavity from the intestinal tissue, thereby increasing pressure within the intestine. Hyperosmotics work fast, between thirty minutes and three hours. **Magnesium sulfate,** an old remedy, is the most potent of them. **Glycerin** works even faster—in fifteen to thirty minutes—but is taken in suppository form. Besides being hyperosmotic, **glycerin** also directly stimulates the colon by local irritation.

There is only one lubricant laxative, **mineral oil.** It works by forming a slippery coat on the interior of the bowel wall to keep the stool moist for easier passage. It also prevents the colon from reabsorbing water and usually works in six to eight hours. It cannot be recommended, however. Although it is the cheapest laxative there is, there are too many problems and potential hazards associated with it.

There is also only one stool softener, **docusate**. It is not actually a laxative; it does not stimulate bowel movements but, rather, helps liquefy the stool by detergent action, causing fat and water to mix together. **Docusate** is used to prevent rather than treat constipation. It is good at helping those who find it difficult or painful to pass hard stool and works in two to three days.

Although most laxatives are taken orally, some, such as **senna**, are also available as suppositories. Enemas, the process of instilling of fluid directly into the rectum, used to be much more popular than they are now. At present, the Fleet enema line is used mainly to prepare patients for diagnostic procedures such as X rays and scoping of the colon.

The main side effects of laxatives are those one would expect: abdominal cramping, excessive gas, and diarrhea. Chronic use can cause continual aggravation of constipation, along with reliance on the drug. Allergies to laxatives are uncommon.

Children and the elderly

Bowel habits vary greatly in children, just as they do in adults, and you should not try to impose your idea of regularity on your child. A good rule to follow is not to give any laxative to a child without instructions from a doctor. Children do not describe symptoms well and what you think may be simple constipation may turn out to be something serious. Acute constipation, for instance, is a sign of appendicitis.

Older adults should be careful of stimulant laxatives. If taken too often they can cause dizziness, lightheadedness, lack of coordination, or weakness.

Pregnancy

Constipation is very common during pregnancy and many women find they need laxatives. The stool softener **docusate** and the bulk forming types are best, but some bulk formers contain a lot of sodium or sugar. Stimulant laxatives, in particular, should be avoided. Nursing mothers should avoid laxatives containing **cascara sagrada** because it may pass into the breast milk. If you are pregnant you should always check with your doctor before using anything.

Other diseases

People with high blood pressure should watch the sodium content of some bulk-forming laxatives. People with diabetes or a weight problem should watch the carbohydrate content of bulk-forming laxatives. People with kidney disease should be careful of hyperosmotic laxatives containing magnesium, potassium, or phosphates.

The magnesium in some hyperosmotic laxatives may interfere with certain medications, such as anticoagulants (blood thinners), heart medications (digitalis), or antibiotics. As a rule, don't take any laxative within two hours of taking any other medicine.

People who are bedridden, have hemorrhoids or other anal diseases, or who have recently had surgery are usually best off with the stool softener **docusate.**

Recommendations

Change your diet to one containing more fiber—what used to be called roughage. High-fiber foods include whole-grain breads, cereals, bran, fruit, and green leafy vegetables. Fruits are particularly good; the old standby, prunes, are excellent. Fiber One has all other cereals beat by a good margin as far as fiber content is concerned, and it contains aspartame (NutraSweet), so it is good for those on a diet. Some people become regular after adding nothing more than an apple a day to their diet. Stay away from sweets and cheese.

Try to retrain yourself if you are chronically constipated. Essentially this means don't suppress the urge to defecate. Welcome it as a call to Nature and respond to it.

Don't take any laxative for more than one week unless your doctor tells you to.

Laxative abuse may lead to dependence. In severe cases this may damage the tissues of the intestines.

Children and adults should be particularly careful with acute constipation, since it can be a sign of appendicitis. Appendicitis in some people is hard to diagnose and people have died of peritonitis because they took laxatives when surgery was indicated.

8

CONTRACEPTIVES

OTC birth-control aids are limited to two methods: condoms and spermicides. They are best used together.

Condoms

There are three types of condoms: latex, polyurethane, and so-called natural. Latex (true rubber) is the cheapest and the best material, and almost all available condoms are made of it. Polyurethane (in the Avanti product line) is a type of plastic, and naturals (under the Fourex and Naturalamb labels) are made of animal membranes. These latter two should be used only by those who are allergic to latex. Symptoms of latex allergy include rash, hives, or wheezing when you come in contact with rubber, as in rubber gloves, balloons, or shower slippers.

The main disadvantage to condoms is that many—possibly most—men don't like them. Women don't care as much. But given the choice between sex with a condom and no sex at all, all men, it is safe to say, will choose the former.

While condoms sometimes fail, studies have shown that the main reason for failure is improper use, often from inexperience.

The rules for condom use are simple:

- Use only fresh latex condoms with a reservoir tip.
- Do not use greasy or oily lubricants. Spermicidal lubricants are best.
- Unroll the condom onto the erect penis before any genital contact takes place.
- As with most things, practice makes perfect.

Contrary to what you might expect, the best time to test for leaks is *after* sex, not before. In other words, don't blow the thing up or fill it with water. Check afterwards. If it appears that the condom has failed, the woman should insert a spermicide, preferably a foam, into the vagina immediately. Foams are best because they act fastest.

Be careful of long fingernails and jewelry when handling condoms.

Condoms are good because they not only protect against pregnancy but also against venereal diseases. They are, in fact, the *only* contraceptive method of any type that also protects against disease, although spermicides do have some minor antiseptic qualities.

Spermicides

Spermicides (vaginal contraceptives) almost all contain the chemical called nonoxynol-9, although one, Ortho-Gynol, contains the almost identical octoxynol-9. Spermicides are designed to be used either by themselves or, better, with a barrier, such as a diaphragm, cervical cap, or condom.

There are five forms of spermicides: foams, creams, jellies, suppositories, and films.

Foams, such as Delfen, Emko, and Koromex, are the most effective forms because of the way they coat the inside of the vagina, but they do not lubricate as well as creams and jellies.

Suppositories and films, both of which have to dissolve in the vaginal secretions, take time to work and are, in general, best avoided.

If you choose a jelly, make sure it is of the proper type. Some are designed to be used by themselves rather than with a diaphragm.

In all cases, follow the manufacturer's directions carefully for specific doses.

The main problem with spermicides is that they have a high failure rate if used by themselves, and so they should be used with a barrier of some sort. If you're going to rely strictly on OTC products, this barrier would be a male condom. Although female condoms are available, they haven't caught on, and they probably never will. They are expensive, ugly, noisy (they squeak), and difficult to use properly, resulting in a high failure rate. All these factors are unfortunate, because medically they make a lot of sense.

Disadvantages to the condom-spermicide combination are that some individuals, men and women, may be allergic to one or more of the ingredients. Even if you are not allergic, frequent use of concentrated spermicides may irritate the vagina or cervix.

Natural methods

The natural methods of birth control are abstinence, rhythm, and ovulation prediction.

Although abstinence is often thought of as the only reliable natural method of birth control, it is impractical. Recommending it is like recommending that people drive at fifty-five miles an hour. In other words, it just won't happen.

The rhythm method is probably the oldest method of birth control for couples. This is how it is done:

A woman keeps track of the length of time between her menstrual periods in days and gathers data over several cycles. The first day of menstrual flow is counted as day number one.

With the numbers in hand, subtract eighteen from the lowest number (shortest length).

Then subtract eleven from the highest number (longest length).

The resulting range is your fertile time.

For example, if your shortest interval between periods is twenty-six days and your longest is thirty days, the time you are fertile is from day eight to day nineteen of your cycle.

Ovulation prediction methods rely on certain body signs to signify fertile times. The basal body temperature method uses the drop in a woman's body temperature shortly before ovulation combined with a rise after ovulation to determine fertility. In the cervical mucus method, women are taught to observe carefully the character of their normal vaginal discharge. Around the time of ovulation the mucus changes from a clear egg-white to a thicker and stickier consistency. A combination of these methods, along with noting mittelschmerz—the lower abdominal discomfort that comes with ovulation—and changes in the tissue of the breasts and labia have also been used, but all are impractical and therefore unreliable.

Birth control is such a personal subject, and one with so many variables, that hard and fast rules are impossible to formulate. Because you have so many choices and because the consequences of unintended pregnancy are so great, it pays to know as much as you can. A sympathetic doctor or family planning clinic is your best bet. You need a prescription for birth control pills or "morning after" pills. Hormonal implants and surgical sterilization are performed by doctors.

Recommendations

Do not rely on withdrawal or douching as methods of birth control. They are too unreliable. Douching promotes vaginal irritation, pelvic infections, and ectopic pregnancies (pregnancies outside of the uterus).

If you are in a stable, monogamous, long-term relationship and do not want to use a surgical, hormonal, or natural method, try a diaphragm or condom and a spermicide. Experiment. Alternate. Use a foam spermicide unless it makes the vagina too dry. In that event try a jelly.

To have "safe" sex with someone you don't know, you should use a latex condom with reservoir tip and impregnated spermicide, along with a spermicidal foam or jelly.

Cost is relative. In all cases, the cost of contraception is infinitely less than the cost of an unintended pregnancy, with or without an abortion, when one takes into account the possibility of complications.

9

DIARRHEA

As with many intestinal disorders, there is no clear cut
definition of diarrhea. It can vary from one or two loose
stools to an almost constant loss of fluid, and in its most
severe forms, such as dysentery or cholera, it can lead to
death. In general, it is a change from customary consistency
that is most significant. Many people have chronically
small, possibly watery bowel movements that for them,
based on diet, physical activity, and constitution, are normal. To others who are used to a firmer stool, any looseness
may be disturbing.

Although diarrhea can have many causes, such as infections, food intolerance, ulcerative colitis, Crohn's disease,
endocrine disease, drugs, and stress, the most helpful first
step in deciding what to do is to determine how long you
have had the problem.

Diarrhea of sudden onset (acute diarrhea)

Diarrhea of this sort is usually infectious, caused by either a
germ or a poison (toxin) produced by a germ. It can start
with a sense of fullness or bloating in the abdomen, loss of
appetite, and excessive gas. One may have headache, fever,
muscle pain, abdominal cramping, nausea, and vomiting.
Stools are usually explosive and very watery.

This type of diarrhea is often borne by foods. It can take
from two to twenty-four hours to develop, depending on the
specific germ. Some, such as *Staphylococcus* (staph) species,
manufacture a poison in the food itself. When the food is
eaten, the toxin works quickly. Others, such as salmonella,

45

which is often found in eggs, work more slowly and cause an actual infection in the intestine. Still others, such as some strains of *E. coli,* both invade the intestine and produce a toxin. Most of the time, the specific germ cannot be discovered. The variation in symptoms is usually not enough to distinguish among them, and medical tests are usually not performed. Even when tests are done, they often turn out to be negative. Besides the organisms listed above, a number of viruses and parasites can be at the root of the problem.

How long the diarrhea lasts also varies. It may be one loose stool or it may persist for weeks, although it is usually over within one to three days.

One way to look at diarrhea is that it is good: your body is trying to get rid of a poison, like draining pus from an abscess. Although when you are sick you don't often think of it this way, the body's response to disease is often beneficial, even when you feel terrible because of it. The most important thing to do with any form of diarrhea, no matter what the cause, is not selecting the most appropriate OTC drug but, rather, making sure you replace the body fluids, nutrients, and electrolytes you are losing.

Balanced fluid replacement is important in anyone with diarrhea, but particularly in children and infants. The younger the child is, the more important this becomes. It doesn't take many watery bowel movements to dehydrate a young tot, with fever and perhaps vomiting adding to the problem. The Centers for Disease Control, in fact, recommends that anyone with children have a supply of fluid and electrolyte replenishing fluid, called oral rehydrating solutions or ORS, on hand. Several of these are available, such as Rehydralyte, Resol, Pedialyte, and Infalyte. Of these, Rehydralyte is the most potent and is indicated for the most effective replenishment of fluids in someone who is already dehydrated.

Infectious diarrhea is different from certain other intestinal problems brought on by foods, such as lactose intolerance. Some people lack the enzyme **lactase** and so have a hard time digesting lactose, the sugar present in milk and ice cream. The sugar makes it all the way to the large intestine, where it causes diarrhea. Experimenting with your diet can help you find out if this is the problem.

Infectious diarrhea may be treatable with prescription antibiotics. Traveller's diarrhea, for example, which is usually caused by *E. coli*-tainted fruits and vegetables, will respond to any of a number of antibiotics, although by the time you get to see a doctor the disease has usually run its three-to-five-day course.

Certain drugs, especially antibiotics, may also cause acute diarrhea. Most antibiotics will produce some alteration in bowel habits but it is usually not serious. In certain cases, however, especially with broad spectrum antibiotics, overgrowth of very toxic intestinal bacteria occur and cause a severe diarrhea. Treatment with another antibiotic must be instituted promptly.

There are no firm rules on when to seek medical attention for acute diarrhea. Most people tough it out, especially if they have been exposed to some bug that is going around. Certainly, however, if you have a very high fever or if the diarrhea lasts more than three days or if there is blood in your stool or if you can't seem to replace the fluids you are losing fast enough because of vomiting or weakness, you should see a doctor.

Chronic diarrhea

How long diarrhea must go on before it is considered chronic is a matter of opinion, but two weeks is about right. Although it may seem incredible, one fairly common cause of chronic diarrhea is overuse of laxatives. This may be the result of emotional problems or child abuse, but it can also be from misguided attempts at weight control. If chronic diarrhea isn't drug related you need a medical evaluation.

Available products

Although there are a number of anti-diarrheals to choose from, one drug, **loperamide** (Imodium and others), clearly stands out as superior. This is because it is easy to take, very effective in all kinds of diarrhea, and has few side effects.

For those who cannot or should not take **loperamide** or for children under six there are two other classes of drugs: adsorbents and **bismuth subsalicylate.**

The adsorbents consist of particles that attract and hold

germs and poisons onto their surfaces. These include **at-tapulgite** (Kaopectate), **kaolin,** and **pectin.** They are not so effective as **loperamide** and are really only good for mild diarrhea. The main disadvantages are that you usually need to take a lot of this kind of product and may find the taste quite unpleasant. Another side effect is that they adsorb not only bad things but good things like nutrients and other medications. If you are taking any prescription medication use adsorbents with caution.

Related to adsorbents is **calcium polycarbophil,** the same product that is used as a bulk-forming laxative. In diarrhea, however, the idea is different. When something *adsorbs* (with a *d)* it causes things to stick to its surface; when it *absorbs* (with a *b)* it actually causes things to be sucked into it. The latter is the case with **calcium polycarbophil;** it will absorb up to sixty times its own weight in water. It is thought to absorb toxic substances along with the water.

Lastly, there is **bismuth subsalicylate** (Pepto-Bismol), which has been around for years and is touted as a virtual panacea for all your intestinal ailments: ". . . the only leading OTC stomach remedy clinically proven effective for both upper and lower GI symptoms." It is labelled as being effective for "upset stomach, indigestion, diarrhea, heart-burn and nausea."

Bismuth subsalicylate can be found in many generic products besides Pepto-Bismol. Often these come in the same type of bottle in the same pink color on the same shelf in the drug store. This drug is in a class by itself. It is a type of salicylate, which means that it is similar to **aspirin.** Although it is often thought of as coating the lining of the stomach, there is actually little evidence that it works this way. It is not an antacid but is used to eradicate (along with antibiotics) the germ *H. pylori,* which is responsible for causing most stomach ulcers. It does have value in preventing and treating certain cases of infectious diarrhea, such as traveller's diarrhea, probably because of its ability to kill some germs, but its use is controversial, and specialists are divided in their opinions about it. Even when used success-fully to treat traveller's diarrhea, the doses needed are far greater than those labelled as safe for OTC use. If you're travelling to a foreign country and are worried, it is best to get your own doctor's advice on what to bring along, if anything. Some doctors will prescribe antibiotics to be taken prophylactically in certain situations.

Recommendations

Don't take an antidiarrheal at the first sign of a loose stool.

The most important thing is to avoid dehydration, particularly in children.

Practice prevention. Wash your hands, the counter top, and utensils after preparing raw meats and fish. Wash the outside of fruits. Refrigerate foods and cook them well. When eating out, avoid eating food that has been standing out at room temperature, such as at buffets.

If your diarrhea is mild and has lasted no more than a week, use **loperamide** for relief of symptoms.

If your diarrhea is more severe or has lasted more than a week, see a doctor.

If you see your doctor, try to be as accurate as you can about the frequency, volume, odor, and character of your bowel movements, along with any other symptoms, such as abdominal pain.

10

DRY VAGINA

Excessive vaginal dryness usually occurs after menopause and is caused by decreased estrogen levels. When severe, there may be burning, itching, and pain upon intercourse. If you are experiencing this and are postmenopausal, consult your doctor for estrogen replacement. Although your age, family history, past history, and general health must be taken into consideration, the great majority of doctors now recommend such therapy. On balance, the benefits outweigh the risks for most patients.

If you are not an estrogen candidate, a number of commercial products are available, such as Astroglide, Feminease, Gyne-Moistrin, H-R Lubricating Jelly, K-Y Jelly, Lubrin Inserts, Maxilube, Moist Again Vaginal Moisturizing, Replens, Surgel, Touch Lubricant, and Women's Health Institute Lubricating gel. They consist of water and ingredients such as **mineral oil, glycerin,** and **propylene glycol,** along with a host of other chemicals. No studies show that one is superior to another, and picking a product that works for you is mostly a matter of trial and error. The standard medical and hospital surgical lubricant for many years has been K-Y Jelly, a water soluble substance containing **glycerin** that is cosmetically pleasing and is easy to remove.

11

EAR PROBLEMS

Problems with the ears can be divided into two groups: those on the skin of the ears themselves, such as rashes, and those inside the ears, such as earaches and hearing loss.

The skin on the ears can be affected by any disease that affects other areas of the skin, such as injuries, eczema, psoriasis, skin cancer, and infections. One common problem is an allergic reaction to earrings, a condition that shows up as redness, scaling, and itching under the earring. This is usually caused by nickel metal in the jewelry. You can experiment to see if this is the case, but you have to understand that allergies of this kind are typically delayed allergies: the rash can start anywhere from one to three days after contact with the offending object. The severity of the eruption also depends upon how long you've worn the earrings and how tightly they fit. Needless to say, the only way to avoid the problem is to avoid the earrings.

Eczema of the ear is also quite common, and is aggravated by the urge to rub and scratch. If you find yourself in one of these itch-scratch cycles, read Chapter 24 (Skin, Hair, and Nails).

Diseases that occur inside the ear canal, on the ear drum, or within the hearing apparatus itself are impossible to diagnose yourself. Not only do they require expertise and special instruments, but even if you were an ear specialist yourself and had the right instruments, you couldn't get a good look inside your own ear.

Thus, if you have an earache, a feeling of fullness in the ear, loss of hearing, ringing in your ears, itching deep inside your ear, bleeding from the ear, discharge from the ear, or you think that a foreign object has become lodged in your ear, you really have to see a doctor about it. Manipulation or irrigation when you don't know what's going on can make matters worse.

There really is only one problem you might consider treating yourself, but only *after* a doctor has told you that this is your problem, and that is excessive ear wax.

Most of the time the ear canal cleans itself, with wax being discharged to the outside, but some people produce large amounts of thick wax that builds up. This can cause diminished hearing as well as a feeling a fullness within the ear.

You or someone at home can help remove wax by gentle irrigation with a soft rubber syringe and **saline** at body temperature, but it is tricky and proper technique is important, so have your doctor tell you if you are a candidate and instruct you on how to do it properly. Don't use Q-tips, paper clips, your fingernails, or your Water Pik. Besides causing injury or introducing bacteria you can actually push the wax deeper into the canal and make it harder to remove. And don't try irrigation if you have ever had a ruptured ear drum, if you have recently had ear surgery, or if you are experiencing dizziness, ear pain, head pain, or drainage.

The only FDA approved active ingredient for ear wax removal at this time is **carbamide peroxide** in **glycerin.** All available commercial products labelled for ear wax removal contain the exact same ingredient in the exact same strength (six and half percent), so that there is little advantage of one over another, although some of them include a soft rubber syringe. Home remedies such as olive oil, **mineral oil,** and **hydrogen peroxide** should be avoided.

There are a number of products, such as Auro-Dri, Dri Ear, Ear-Dry, and Swim-Ear, whose names might lead you to believe that they are good for water in the ear canals. They contain nothing more than **alcohol,** however, as their main ingredient. Although **alcohol** is a good antiseptic, these products are of questionable value. If you have water in your ear, let it drain out by gravity.

12

EYE PROBLEMS

Eye disorders that can be suitably treated with OTC products include dry eyes, red eyes, itchy eyes, and some disorders of the eyelids. Many eye products should only be used for short periods—a few days at the most—unless being used for dry eyes or contact lenses; overusing eye drops can aggravate your condition. If your symptoms are severe and include intense eye pain, head pain, or blurred vision, delay in seeking treatment can be very dangerous. On the other hand, if you get some toxic or irritating liquid in your eyes, immediate irrigation of your eyes with water or **saline** may save your sight. Obviously, if you are at all unsure of the seriousness of your problem, seek medical attention promptly.

Dry eyes

Dry eyes are a very common problem, especially in older women. Most often they are caused by low humidity in the environment, the result of air conditioning or heated rooms, but dry eyes can also result from cosmetic surgery that prevents the lids from closing properly. Some drugs, such as antihistamines, antidepressants, diuretics (water pills), and beta blockers (heart medications) can be the cause of dryness. Autoimmune diseases, in which the immune system reacts against the body's own tissues, can create the same problem. This is especially true of rheumatoid arthritis.

Dry eyes may not actually feel dry but may burn or itch. The whites of your eyes may or may not be red.

The available OTC preparations for dry eyes are commonly called artificial tears. Ointments (greases), however, are also available for nighttime use, since tear production is lowered when sleeping. If your eyes are very dry you may have to use artificial tears as often as every hour, but even this may be insufficient, and doctors sometimes treat severely dry eyes by blocking the tear ducts (which are drains) to preserve one's own tear production.

The ingredients found in artificial tear products are often the same as those used in other eye preparations as solvents or vehicles for the delivery of actual drugs. Artificial tears can thus be considered non-medicated eye drops.

Ingredients in liquid artificial tears are often called demulcents, which are substances that coat, protect, and lubricate mucous membranes. These include **cellulose ethers,** dextran, **glycerin, polyvinyl alcohol, propylene glycol,** gelatin, **polyethylene glycol** (300 and 400), polysorbate 80, and **povidone,** all of which are roughly equivalent. The ointments contain combinations of **mineral oil, petrolatum,** and **lanolin.** Both types are usually safe to use.

Most of these products contain preservatives (antiseptics)—substances that kill germs. Included in artificial tears are such chemicals as **sodium edetate, benzalkonium chloride, sorbic acid, sodium borate,** and **boric acid.** Although these are usually present in very small concentrations, some people are sensitive to them, especially those who must instill the drops frequently. Preservative-free preparations have been devised to counteract this problem, but since they come in tiny containers that can be used only once or a few times, they are more expensive. If you use such a product more than once, it is best to keep it in a refrigerator to prevent bacterial growth once it has been opened. If you need artificial tears regularly, make a note of the preservative or preservatives that are in the solution. If your eyes become irritated, it may be less expensive to switch to a product with different preservatives rather than go to a completely preservative-free product.

Red eyes

The eyes can become itchy, teary, and red for a variety of reasons, such as injuries, foreign bodies, dust, chemicals, allergies, and dryness. There may be an associated burning feeling. More serious conditions, such as infections, can also cause red eyes.

The conjunctiva is the delicate tissue that lines the inside of the eyelids and covers the white portion of your eye. Inflammation of this tissue—the main symptom of which is redness—is called conjunctivitis. People often call this pink eye, and it may be caused by any number of things.

Conjunctivitis, like inflammation elsewhere, has a certain protective function. The redness is due to dilated blood vessels, which act to bring in beneficial blood cells and to carry away toxic materials. Tearing may also be increased and serves to wash out and dilute noxious substances. Tears also contain substances that may inhibit germs.

Conjunctivitis caused by a virus may be highly contagious, and care should be taken to avoid spreading it to other family members or co-workers. Although viral conjunctivitis clears up by itself and there is no specific medical treatment, prescription medications may relieve some of the symptoms. It may, however, be very difficult to distinguish it from bacterial conjunctivitis, a condition that can be treated with prescription antibiotics. You should see a doctor as soon as possible if your red eyes are associated with pain, pus, thick discharge, sensitivity to light, or the feeling that there is something in your eye. Also see a doctor if you have red eyes and wear contact lenses.

Allergic conjunctivitis is often associated with nasal stuffiness and discharge in the typical hay fever pattern of symptoms. The eyes, nose, and sometimes the roof of the mouth may itch. There may be associated asthma, eczema, and hives. Referring to Chapter 1 (Allergies) may be helpful.

Red eyes may be associated with blepharitis. Blepharitis is inflammation—redness, swelling, and often scaling—of the eyelid or its margins. This condition is often associated with excessive and inflammatory dandruff of the scalp (seborrhea) or with adult acne (rosacea). It is important to know that in children, blepharitis may be a sign of lice, in which case the insects and their eggs (nits) can be seen on the eyelashes.

Blepharitis may predispose one to the formation of styes, which are infections of the eyelid glands. These may occur on the inner portion or the outer portion of the lids, and although tending to resolve spontaneously, they may linger for weeks or months. Since some styes may be due to bacteria that respond to antibiotics, it is generally wise to seek medical attention promptly.

Redness, swelling, scaling, and itching of the skin on the eyelid itself (not at the margins where the eyelashes grow) is often secondary to some type of eczema or contact allergy, and although **hydrocortisone** in cream or ointment form can be used for treatment, it is much better to have your condition accurately diagnosed by your doctor before embarking on a course of this topical steroid.

There are four OTC active ingredients for red eyes, all of which are decongestants: **naphazoline, tetrahydrozoline, oxymetazoline,** and **phenylephrine.** As with the decongestants used in cough, cold, and allergy products, they work by constricting or narrowing blood vessels. This reduces the redness.

As with nasal decongestants, however, you have to watch out for rebound, in which redness, swelling, and tearing are produced by the medications themselves. This tends to occur more frequently in those who overuse eye drops.

As a rule, products containing **naphazoline** in at least a .02 percent concentration have been shown to be somewhat more effective than other preparations and have a decreased tendency to produce rebound.

Some products combine the antihistamines **pheniramine** and **antazoline** with **naphazoline** but list the antihistamines as inactive ingredients. This is because the FDA considers them to be ineffective, but this position is controversial, and some studies show that antihistamines do indeed reduce red eye symptoms. On the other hand, they can cause stinging in some individuals, and if you are allergic to them, they will aggravate your condition.

Taking the above into consideration, the most useful OTC medications for red eyes are the ones that are free of antihistamine and contain at least .02 percent **naphazoline.** Product names fulfilling these requirements include Sensitive Eyes Redness Reliever Lubricant Maximum Strength and VasoClear. Similar products *with* antihistamines are Naphcon A, OcuHist, Opcon-A, and Vaso-con-A.

Swelling of the cornea

The FDA allows high concentrations (two percent and five percent) of **saline** to be sold OTC. These products, called hyperosmotics, are indicated for swelling of the cornea, the medical term for which is corneal edema. Although this condition may be caused by contact lenses that fit poorly or are worn for extended periods, the use of hyperosmotics is usually confined to more chronic conditions, such as Fuchs' dystrophy. Symptoms of swelling of the cornea include light sensitivity, blurring of vision, and seeing halos, starbursts, or rainbows around lights. Your eye may also feel hot, itchy, or gritty. It should go without saying that these symptoms should prompt you to see your doctor. If a **saline** hyperosmotic is recommended, you won't need a prescription to get one. The five percent product tends to sting when applied.

Eye washes

These are also known as eye irrigants, and are most useful in emergencies to flush harmful chemicals or foreign bodies out of the eye, although they can also be used to cleanse away mucus or pus in cases of infection. They should not be used with contact lenses because of the preservatives they contain and because they disrupt the composition of tears. An excellent eye irrigant is **saline** (.9 percent), but water can be used in an emergency if **saline** is not available. Eye cups, which are sometimes sold with these products, are not recommended because they can easily become contaminated. Commercial OTC eye irrigants other than plain **saline** usually contain a combination of salts, preservatives, and chemical buffers to make them soothing and germ free. There is no clear advantage to these over plain **saline** used as described above.

Astringents

Astringents have two main effects: they cause contraction of tissue and they precipitate protein. Ocular astringents are mostly designed to perform the latter function, in order to precipitate the protein portion of a mucus discharge out of solution and cause it to clump. The most common of these ingredients is **zinc sulfate** and it is incorporated in several preparations. The FDA allows the following labelling for astringents: "For the temporary relief of discomfort from minor eye irritations." These products are best avoided unless your doctor has recommended one.

Contact lens products

There are three types of contact lenses, hard, gas permeable, and soft. Each type, in turn, is subdivided into lenses with varying characteristics. The advantages and disadvantages of each type of lens are beyond the scope of this book, but because they are easy to use and safe, soft lenses are used most frequently.

There are two steps necessary in caring for most contact lenses: cleaning and storing. Each lens type has its own recommendations for care, often with its own lens care product line. Using certain lenses properly can consume both time and money, and studies have shown that most people are careless in adhering to the advised routines. Difficulties arise most often not from poor products but from poor care.

Drug stores devote considerable shelf space to lens care products. As a rule, the best way to insure safety is to follow the manufacturer's instructions to the letter. In particular, do not mix products from different manufacturers, since they often use different preservatives, and some of them may actually cause precipitates when mixed with each other. Similarly, do not try to mix salt tablets with tap water to make your own saline; these are unsterile solutions and sight threatening infections have resulted from such concoctions.

It is also important to take out your lenses if you are applying eye drops, unless they are the rewetting drops specifically designed for your lenses. Rewetting drops are designed to make water adhere better to the lens surface and to provide lubrication and cushioning.

Recommendations

Don't try to treat any eye injury unless it is very minor.

OTC products are not meant to cure eye infections, but only to relieve symptoms.

Don't use any OTC for more than a few days unless your doctor recommends otherwise.

13

FEVER

Body temperature is one of the most important pieces of information you can have about yourself. It is usually constant, easily and accurately measured, and gives a good indication of how healthy or sick you are. It can also be used to monitor treatment for a disease and to predict recovery from that disease. A fever means that something is wrong.

Chills are sometimes associated with fevers. Medically, doctors make a distinction between simply feeling cold or chilly, which is seen in just about all fevers, and the type of chill in which your teeth chatter.

Although fever therapy was once the rage for various illnesses, there is little evidence that an elevated temperature does us much good when we are sick. The slight increase of a few degrees really isn't enough to make much of a difference in how well the immune system is able to fight off infections or otherwise repair damaged tissue. On the other hand, there is ample evidence of the harmful effects of fever. Besides making us feel terrible, a high fever makes the heart work harder and the resulting perspiration causes us to lose water and electrolytes. It also uses up nutrients at an accelerated rate because of the increase in metabolism.

There are different definitions of what exactly constitutes a fever, but an oral temperature of 100.4° F (38° C) is generally about right, although some specialists put the figure at 100° F. The higher the number is above this, of course, the more serious the problem. Rectal temperatures run about two degrees (F) above the oral. There is great variation in armpit (axillary) measurements, and skin strips that change color are almost entirely unreliable. The newer electronic thermometers, which measure infrared radiation from the ear canal, however, are very accurate and very fast, but cost considerably more than the old standby mercury-and-glass devices. Still, if you have young children, it may be worthwhile to have one on hand. Directions should be followed carefully to get the best readings.

Table 5. Temperature conversion

Centigrade (C)	Fahrenheit (F)
36°	96.8°
37°	98.6°
38°	100.4°
39°	102.2°
40°	104°
41°	105.8°

Most fevers are caused by infections with germs (bacteria and viruses most commonly), but there are many other possibilities, including medications, cancer, heart attacks, an overactive thyroid, serious injuries, strokes, autoimmune diseases—in which the immune system reacts against the body's own tissues—and even gout. Dehydration may lead to fever in infants but it is rarely the cause in adults.

Fever sometimes occurs for no detectable reason. The condition known as fever of unknown origin (FUO) can be one of the most baffling challenges in medicine. It is generally defined as a fever that lasts for more than two to three weeks in which all diagnostic tests are within normal limits.

Small elevations of temperature do not need to be treated at all. Some people are not overly bothered by the slight feeling of warmth, and treating a fever sometimes causes excessive perspiration and chills. Treatment becomes mandatory, however, when the fever becomes a problem in its own right or when there is heart failure, mental confusion, a tendency toward seizures, or heat stroke. *If you have recently had a surgical operation or invasive medical test, call your doctor immediately to report any elevation in temperature and make no attempt to treat it on your own.*

The medications that reduce fever are all internal analgesics, and discussion of them can be found in Chapter 22 on pain. In general, avoid **aspirin** in anyone under the age of sixteen because of the risk of precipitating the serious disease known as Reye's syndrome. **Acetaminophen** (Tylenol) remains the safest antipyretic (fever reducer) for everyone, but the NSAIDs **ibuprofen, ketoprofen,** and **naproxen** are also effective. A special pediatric **ibuprofen** product is available (Children's Motrin).

These drugs should always be taken in a steady and regular dose. If you wait for the temperature to go up too high, you can precipitate chills and sweating. This is not dangerous in itself but can be extremely uncomfortable. If the temperature goes much above 104° F (40° C), lukewarm baths or towel compresses should be instituted. Avoid ice compresses and do not apply alcohol. Fluids, which are important to anyone with a fever, become crucial when the temperature is this high.

14

FIRST AID

OTC products for first aid are mainly designed for minor injuries—scrapes, cuts, burns, and puncture wounds. In addition, there are products for treating certain cases of poisoning. We will discuss injuries first.

At the outset, you have to remember that the marvellous thing about the human body is that it tends to heal itself. All living creatures possess a certain ability to repair themselves. They don't have to think about it most of the time and they don't have to do anything special to bring it about. Indeed, throughout most of history we did not have Band-Aids, antibiotics, drugstores, or doctors of any sort. So if you injure yourself and do nothing you can expect the injury to be repaired in some way within a week or two. There may be evidence of that injury in the form of a scar or discoloration, but the wound itself will be gone. In some areas of the body, such as the mouth, the healing is wonderfully fast. If you bite your cheek or tongue, for instance, no matter how deep or painful it is you're usually not even aware of it a couple of days later.

This is assuming that you are otherwise healthy. People with diabetes, circulation problems, malnutrition, or immune deficiencies may not heal as well, and in some severe cases of debilitation, healing never does take place.

The first thing to do with any injury is to determine how bad it is. If it is gaping, bleeding profusely, or has reached the level of muscle, tendon, or bone, obviously, you should seek emergency care. The same goes if you haven't received a tetanus shot in some time. It is suggested that tetanus boosters be given every five years if an injury has been sustained.

For a wound that is actively bleeding, direct pressure with a clean piece of gauze is still the best treatment. Don't dab and look every few seconds; keep the pressure on for a full five minutes by the clock. If the bleeding hasn't stopped, try again for another five minutes. If it is still bleeding after two tries, you should seek professional help; you'll probably need some stitches.

For cleaning almost any wound, soap and water is fine. If it is convenient, allow fresh running water to flow over the area. Puncture wounds should be soaked in warm soapy water. **Saline,** if available, is good for irrigation because it is gentle and doesn't sting, but it is not essential.

Once the wound is clean you should place a suitable dressing on it and change it daily. Adhesive bandages come in various sizes, and one should be selected that covers all edges adequately. For large abrasions you will have to devise a dressing yourself with pieces of sterile gauze and tape. Some people are very allergic to the adhesives on bandages and tape, however, and it is not uncommon to develop more trouble from tape than from the wound itself. Paper tapes are kinder and gentler in this regard, but they don't stick as well.

What to put on the wound, around the wound, and on the bandage—if anything—is a matter of some controversy. Many studies have been done in an attempt to find out how best to speed healing and prevent infection, but there continues to be disagreement on some of the details. Everyone agrees, though, that you should try to do two things:

- Prevent infection
- Keep the wound moist

Preventing infection

There are two broad classes of OTC substances that can help prevent infection: antiseptics and antibiotics. An antiseptic is something (usually a chemical of some sort) that will kill just about any germ. An antibiotic is something (usually a biological product produced by a yeast or fungus) that will kill only certain germs, namely bacteria.

There are many different types of germs: bacteria, viruses, fungi, and parasites. Each type may have dozens of subtypes, and each of these, in turn, has its own personality. Some like it warm, others prefer it cool; some thrive in the presence of oxygen, others die in the presence of oxygen; some like it moist, and some like it dry. And some cause disease, whereas others prevent disease.

This last characteristic is very important: not all germs are bad. Most, in fact, are very good. They aid in Nature's recycling, they help in digestion, and they provide an essential balance without which life would be impossible. If it were not for germs we would be inundated with waste products and dead bodies that would not decompose. We need germs, in other words, more than they need us.

Germs have a bad reputation because of the few of them that cause human disease. It would be good if we could be very selective and eliminate only these, but it is very difficult. Microorganisms, although different in many respects, do share some fundamental biological processes, and this is where the difference between antiseptics and antibiotics comes in.

Most antiseptics are based on the principle that if a chemical is strong enough it will act like a poison and kill just about anything. Most antibiotics, however, are based on the principle that the two largest groups of germs, fungi (or molds) and bacteria, are natural enemies. The molds produce substances that tend to kill only bacteria.

The difference between antiseptics and antibiotics is important for this reason: bacteria tend to develop resistance to antibiotics but not to antiseptics. Much of the criticism levelled at the medical profession for the overuse of antibiotics might also be levelled at any consumer who applies an antibiotic ointment to a cut or scrape that is otherwise clean. Although the antibiotic might prevent infection, it might also be causing new and more deadly bacteria to arise.

As a practical matter, however, externally applied antibiotics are in very widespread use throughout medicine. Three of them are available OTC: **bacitracin, neomycin,** and **polymyxin B.** These are produced in various combinations, often as triple antibiotic ointments. Each antibiotic is effective against different types of bacteria, but they have no effect whatsoever on viruses or other types of germs. The combinations have generally been selected so that they cover a wide spectrum of bacteria. Antibiotic ointments are generally well tolerated, except for **neomycin,** which sometimes causes severe allergic skin irritation. This irritation can look a lot like infection, and it is not uncommon for someone to seek medical attention for a persistent wound infection that turns out to be a medication allergy. To avoid this, a combination that includes only **bacitracin** and **polymyxin B,** such as Polysporin, is safest.

Antibiotic ointments can be applied generously directly to the wound and to the skin around a wound or to the bandage itself. On the scalp, a thick coating can actually substitute for a bandage, which is difficult to apply because of the hair.

When deciding whether you want to use an antibiotic or an antiseptic, it is important to understand that antiseptics, unlike antibiotics, are designed to be used only on *intact* skin, not on open wounds themselves. Thus, they can be used before surgery, or to disinfect the hands before handling food, or around wounds. When applied within a wound the harsh chemicals can actually kill cells and delay healing.

The FDA has developed a complicated system for classifying antiseptics into four categories depending on their intended use, such as skin preparation before surgery, hand cleansing among food handlers, and personal use in the home. Each antiseptic ingredient may be present in more than one category, but the labels are different. Among the approved individual antiseptics are **alcohol, benzalkonium chloride, benzethonium chloride, chlorhexidine, hexylresorcinol, hydrogen peroxide, iodine, povidone-iodine, methylbenzethonium chloride,** and **phenol.** Two combinations are also approved: **camphor** and **phenol,** and **eucalyptol, menthol, methylsalicylate,** and **thymol.** This last concoction, by the way, is what is in Listerine antiseptic, which is only for use as a mouthwash.

There is a way to simplify matters, because only two of these ingredients, **alcohol** and **povidone-iodine,** are approved for use in all four categories. For general use, then, either one is satisfactory. **Alcohol** is inexpensive, freely available, and a very good all-around antiseptic. If overused, however, it can dry out the skin. **Povidone-iodine,** the best known brand of which is Betadine, is more expensive. The other antiseptics have little in their favor for first-aid use. **Hydrogen peroxide** in particular, although time honored and cheap, has a tendency to damage healing tissue.

Keeping it moist

Studies have shown that wounds heal faster if they are kept from drying out. Perhaps people could learn something from the instinctive behavior of wounded animals, who lick their wounds. Why do they do this? To apply some natural antibiotic or antiseptic present in their saliva? Not at all. Although saliva contains enzymes and other substances that promote healing, there are also loads of bacteria in there. Animals lick their wounds to keep them moist and to rid them of dirt and other foreign bodies. So keeping injured skin moist—as long as it is free from infection—is a good idea. This is another advantage to topical antibiotics, which usually come in ointment (greasy) form.

Although an antibiotic ointment under a plain gauze dressing is probably as good a treatment as any for minor injuries, a thriving industry has grown up around new and improved wound coverings designed solely to prevent drying while allowing for the circulation of oxygen and carbon dioxide. Among these are thin plastic films or jelly-like substances such as Op-Site, Tegaderm, ACU-derm, Uniflex, Kaltostat, Sorbsan, Elasto-Gel, Vigilon, and Viasorb. There are others with different features. They work well, reduce pain, and have many advantages over traditional dressings, but they are expensive. They are probably not warranted for injuries you are likely to take care of by yourself, but for more extensive wounds your doctor may use or recommend one to good advantage.

Two alternatives to plain dry gauze are nonadherent dressings such as Telfa and **petrolatum**-impregnated dressings like Adaptic. At least one study has shown that **petrolatum** (petroleum jelly) compares very favorably to more expensive antibiotic ointments as a covering for wounds; infection rates for the two groups are almost equal. If a wound is not infected and has not been subject to contamination, a simple dressing with **petrolatum** is a reasonable choice.

Minor burns

The care of small superficial burns is similar to that for other injuries, except that as initial first aid you should run cold water over the affected area for several minutes in order to reduce the chance of a blister.

As long as the skin stays intact there is little danger of infection. One of the FDA approved protectants, such as **allantoin, cocoa butter, petrolatum,** or **shark liver oil** may be applied. **Hydrocortisone** ointment serves the same purpose and may provide some reduction in pain. Local anesthetics tend to be too weak and of too short a duration to provide much relief. Household butter, similarly, is ineffective.

If the skin is broken take measures to prevent infection and keep the area moist. *Do not use hydrocortisone on an open area of skin, since it can promote infection.*

If the burn seems to be more than you are comfortable handling, seek medical attention. This applies particularly to burns from electrical shocks, since they are usually deeper than they seem.

Eye injuries

If you accidently get some chemical or toxic liquid in your eye an immediate flushing with **saline** or water can save your sight. The general treatment is immediate irrigation coupled with a call to the doctor. As a general rule you should continue to flush for twenty minutes, then head off to the emergency room or doctor's office.

Foreign bodies present a special problem. If they are small your own tears will usually wash them out, but the larger ones need medical attention. If you play squash, shoot guns, mow the lawn with a power mower, work with wood, or participate in other activities, hobbies, or sports that can create projectiles, you can prevent problems by wearing eye guards.

15

GAS

Excess gas means different things to different people. To one, it may be flatus (farting), while to another it may be belching or bloating, pressure, cramping, or fullness and discomfort in the abdomen. It's important to understand that the feeling of discomfort may actually have nothing whatever to do with gas, unless you are clearly relieved by expelling it. It is also important to understand that to a certain degree, passing rectal gas is not only perfectly normal, but is linked to a healthy diet.

The FDA actually classifies foods according to how much intestinal gas they produce. Foods that produce gas are called flatulogenic. High gas producers include beans, bagels, bran, broccoli, brussels sprouts, cabbage, cauliflower, and onions. More moderate gas producers include apples, apricots, bananas, bread, carrots, celery, citrus fruits, eggplant, lettuce, pastries, radishes, raisins, and prune juice.

The reason these foods cause flatulence is because they contain high amounts of undigestible sugars that are transported to the large intestine and are fermented by the bacteria found there. The fermentation produces simpler sugars and carbon dioxide, methane, and hydrogen. Beans, because of the sugars stachyose and raffinose, are particularly effective in this regard.

This is the rationale behind the use of Beano, which contains **alpha-galactosidase,** an enzyme that breaks down the complex sugars to more simple ones that can be digested in the stomach before intestinal bacteria can get to them. For this reason you have to take the Beano along with the food you predict will give you trouble. In other words, if you wait until the farting begins, it's too late. Although the enzyme is used in food processing and is found in small amounts in many foods, Beano contains more of it. Since it is derived from a mold, those with mold allergies may develop allergic symptoms. Those with diabetes should also be careful, since the enzyme tends to produce more digestable sugar from foods than would normally be the case. Finally, those with the rare genetic enzyme deficiency disease called galactosemia cannot use Beano.

Gas can also be produced by lactose. Lactose is a sugar present in milk and other dairy products. Normally, the enzyme **lactase** converts lactose into ordinary sugar. People who are deficient in this enzyme have trouble with the conversion and develop gas, diarrhea, bloating, and cramps after ingesting dairy products. The diagnosis can be proved by means of a lactose tolerance test but you can confirm it yourself by keeping a careful record of your diet and symptoms. By staying away from dairy products for several days, then ingesting milk, you can reproduce for yourself the symptoms of lactose intolerance if they exist.

People who swallow air or who drink carbonated beverages, such as soft drinks, beer, or champagne, may be prone to gas purely from ingesting too much of it. Ill fitting dentures, chewing gum, and diet candies or mints may also cause one to swallow air, as may using a straw to drink liquids. In some individuals, air swallowing is an unconscious habit. The usual symptom is belching.

The most widely used OTC drug for gas is **simethicone**, but its effectiveness is controversial. Indeed, one advisory panel to the FDA came to the conclusion that it was effective, whereas another did not, and the final result was that the FDA went with the first recommendation.

Many antacids contain **simethicone** as an added ingredient, but there is little actual evidence that the combination is of any value, since the indications for the antacid are not the same as the indications for the gas. Furthermore, one study revealed that **simethicone** added to an antacid containing aluminum reduced the efficacy of both substances.

If you really are troubled by gas you can buy **simethicone** alone in the form of tablets, capsules, or liquid, such as Phazyme or Silain. **Simethicone** is very safe since it is an inert substance that is not absorbed into the bloodstream and has no known side effects. There are some preparations of it that are designed for infants and children with colic. Since children have a hard time describing symptoms, it is debatable whether a crying infant is indeed suffering from excess gas. Still, **simethicone** is safe, so that if your pediatrician recommends it, it may be worth a try. The real question is not the safety or effectiveness of **simethicone** in children but whether you may be missing a more serious abdominal problem.

Activated charcoal, although not approved by the FDA for intestinal gas, has some strong proponents. The usual dose, however, and the way it should be prepared (as a gritty sludge) make it highly unpalatable. At least one product (Flatulex) contains both **simethicone** and **activated charcoal** in a more acceptable form.

Recommendations

If you are having abdominal symptoms, try to be specific about the problem: is it a feeling of fullness or bloating? Of pain? Of belching? Of flatulence—excess gas passed through the rectum? It is only the last which is properly termed gas.

Avoid carbonated beverages, chewing gum, and diet candies. Don't drink through a straw. Get your dentures fitted properly and be aware if you are swallowing air.

If this fails and you're planning a party that features cabbage and bean soup, try Beano.

16

HEARTBURN, ACID INDIGESTION, AND SOUR STOMACH

Abdominal problems can be very tricky to diagnose, and even specialists can have a hard time with them. If you take medication without the benefit of medical advice you only have your symptoms to guide you, and symptoms in the abdominal cavity can be notoriously hard to interpret. Furthermore, one of the most common symptoms, heartburn, isn't abdominal pain but chest pain, so that there is the added possibility that your heart may be the source of it.

The symptoms for which OTC products are designed are usually labelled "heartburn, acid indigestion, and sour stomach," which some people refer to as an upset stomach. But the common denominator for all of them is either too much stomach acid or stomach acid where it shouldn't be, namely in the esophagus, the tube which runs from your throat to your stomach.

Heartburn is a symptom most people have had at some point in their lives. The frequency and degree of discomfort vary greatly, with some individuals experiencing it only rarely and mildly, while others have it so often that it interferes with work and sleep. Pregnant woman often suffer from it frequently. As its name implies, it is a burning pain that occurs in the center of the lower chest, beneath the breast bone, although it can radiate throughout the chest, back, and into the throat. It has nothing to do with the heart but is caused by regurgitation of acidic and irritating stomach contents upwards into the esophagus.

Acid indigestion is a more vague complaint, and many cases of it have turned out to be fatal heart attacks.

Sour stomach refers to that unpleasant sensation and awful taste when the acid and partially digested food regurgitates and travels all the way up into the back of your throat or mouth. This is also called water brash.

Normally, the upward movement of stomach contents is prevented by a muscular band of tissue located at the junction of the esophagus and stomach called the lower esophageal sphincter. Some people have a weak sphincter or one that is prone to frequent relaxations. Then, because of pressure within the stomach, contents are forced upwards, irritating the sensitive tissues in the esophagus. The esophagus, unlike the stomach, is not designed for acid.

If this happens once in a while it is nothing more than an annoyance, but if it becomes chronic and goes on for years, the tissue of the esophagus can be permanently damaged, and the condition may even lead to cancer. There is also a type of asthma that is triggered by it. The medical term for these symptoms or changes is gastroesophageal reflux disease or GERD.

Before deciding which drug is best if you have GERD you should know that there are many things you can do to reduce your symptoms without medications of any kind.

Adjust your diet. Stay away from hot spicy foods and alcohol. Also avoid fats, citrus juices, and coffee.

Reduce the size of your meals and avoid lying down right after a meal. Enjoy your last meal of the day at least three hours before going to bed.

Many people suffer most or exclusively at night or when they recline. This makes sense, since the effects of gravity are reduced. If this is the case, raise the head of your bed with blocks under the end of it.

Stop smoking. It increases stomach acid.

If you are overweight, try to lose weight and avoid tight-fitting clothing, which increase pressure within the abdomen.

Some people have a habit of swallowing air. This also increases pressure within the stomach. Avoid chewing gum and carbonated beverages for this reason.

If you are taking medications such as hormones, high blood pressure medications, tranquilizers, or antidepressants, check with your doctor or look them up in a suitable drug reference to see if they tend to promote heartburn. Certain drugs relax the esophageal sphincter.

If these measures don't help you can choose between two forms of OTC therapy, antacids, which neutralize existing stomach acid, and HRAs (histamine H_2-receptor antagonists), which reduce its production. At the present time there is an advertising slugfest going on between the manufacturers of each type, who are competing for your GERD dollar. At the very simplest level, the following can be said about these products: although they both help, the antacids work much faster, within minutes, whereas the the HRAs take an hour or two. The HRAs, however, help for hours.

Antacids

There are well over a hundred individual antacid products from which to choose, but as the partial list of them in Table 6 shows, there are only four basic classes of active ingredients: sodium, calcium, **magnesium,** and aluminum salts. Each antacid ingredient has its pros and cons, and they are often mixed to balance these out.

Sodium bicarbonate, such as is found in ordinary baking soda and Alka Seltzer, has great neutralizing capacity and acts almost at once, but contains huge amounts of sodium. This can be dangerous for those on a sodium restricted diet, and isn't good in any event. It is also the only antacid that is completely absorbed and that can change the acidity of the blood. Thus, it should be used, if at all, only in very limited amounts for very short periods of time.

Calcium carbonate, the substance found in Tums (and chalk), is also a good acid neutralizer, but works more slowly, although its effect is more prolonged. About ten percent of the calcium is absorbed. Despite the hoopla about increasing one's calcium intake, too much isn't good for you, particularly if your kidneys aren't working properly.

Magnesium salts such as **magnesium hydroxide, magnesium oxide, magnesium carbonate,** and **magnesium trisilicate**

are somewhat weaker antacids than the above but tend to produce diarrhea. Because of absorption of magnesium, however, they should be used with great caution if you have kidney disease.

Aluminum salts such as **aluminum hydroxide** and **aluminum carbonate** have the weakest neutralizing capacity. If your kidneys are functioning normally, any excess aluminum will be excreted, but if they are not, elevated aluminum levels can result. In addition, too much aluminum antacid reduces the amount of phosphate from your intestine. But the most common side effect is constipation, which can be severe.

In order to minimize the side effects of constipation and diarrhea, many popular antacids combine ingredients, most commonly **aluminum hydroxide** and one of the magnesium salts. Magaldrate, one of the most popular of these, is a mixture of **aluminum hydroxide** and **magnesium hydroxide**. A few antacids even combine these two with **calcium carbonate** and **sodium bicarbonate**. Whether or not these concoctions are better is questionable. With regard to the constipation-diarrhea issue, most combinations still tend to produce diarrhea, the magnesium component outweighing the aluminum.

The strength of a particular antacid product depends on factors other than composition. Suspensions, for example, are generally more effective and work faster than tablets. Some companies provide information on neutralizing capacity by providing a number, called the acid neutralizing capacity (ANC). The higher the number, the greater the capacity, and the stronger the product. The only way to make an accurate comparison between antacids is to know this number. Unfortunately, a high ANC doesn't necessarily mean that a product is pleasant tasting or devoid of side effects. How well antacids work also depends upon how you take them. They have the longest duration (up to three hours) if taken about an hour after you eat, but they last only about thirty minutes if taken on a completely empty stomach.

Sodium bicarbonate and **calcium carbonate** can cause the rebound effect, in which acidity returns to an even higher level after you stop using them. Too much of any of these products can contribute to a disease known as the milk-alkali syndrome, the symptoms of which are headache, irritability, weakness, and nausea. In its later stages kidney disease can result.

Because antacids reduce stomach acid, they can upset the natural processes of digestion and interfere with the absorption of many medications. The most well known of these problems are interactions with antibiotics, particularly the tetracyclines, but the effectiveness of other medications that may be taken for the digestion, such as HRAs (see below) and sucralfate (a prescription medicine for ulcers), may also be impaired. Changed absorption may also occur when taking **aspirin,** allopurinol, anticonvulsants, or ketoconazole, and heart medications such as beta blockers, digoxin, and quinidine. As a rule, don't take any oral medications within two hours of an antacid, unless your doctor tells you otherwise.

If you are a diabetic you should be aware that many antacids contain sugar. If you are ingesting large quantities for an extended period, it may make a difference in your condition.

Some antacids, such as Gaviscon, advertise that they float on the surface of the stomach contents, so that any regurgitated material is actually the antacid itself. They do this by including **alginic acid** along with the antacid. However, you won't see **alginic acid** listed as an active ingredient because, although there are some studies that bear out the claim, the FDA still questions its efficacy. In any event, if it does work, it only works if you are standing upright. It is not effective when you are lying down, which is when much heartburn occurs.

Pepto-Bismol **(bismuth subsalicylate),** the panacea for all sorts of intestinal complaints, has been around for a long time, and is in a class by itself. Although labelled for heartburn, it is not an antacid, does not neutralize stomach acid, and probably does not coat your stomach lining. In some respects, however, it is a very interesting and potentially valuable drug. It is discussed in Chapter 9 on diarrhea.

Table 6. Antacids

Brand	Aluminum salt	Magnesium salt	Calcium carbonate	Sodium bicarbonate
Acid-X			X	
Alka-Mints			X	
Alka-Seltzer caplets & gelcaps	X			
Alka-Seltzer effervescent tablets				X
Alkets			X	
Almora		X		
AlternaGEL	X			
Amitone			X	
Amphojel	X			
Arm & Hammer Baking Soda				X
Basaljel	X			
Bell/ans				X
Bromo-Seltzer				X
Chooz			X	
Citrocarbonate				X
Creamalin	X	X		
Dialume	X			
Di-Gel liquid	X	X		
Di-Gel tablet		X	X	
Dicarbosil			X	
Equilet			X	
Gaviscon	X	X		X
Gelusil	X	X		
Genelac			X	
Kudrox	X	X		
Losopan	X	X		
Maalox suspension	X	X		
Maalox caplets		X	X	
Marblen		X	X	
Milk of magnesia		X		
Mylanta	X	X		
Mylanta Lozenges			X	

Brand	Aluminum salt	Magnesium salt	Calcium carbonate	Sodium bicarbonate
Nephrox	X			
Phillips' Chewable		X		
Riopan	X	X		
Simaal	X	X		
Tempo	X	X	X	
Titralac			X	
Tums			X	

Histamine receptor antagonists (HRAs)

Histamine is a potent, naturally occurring chemical that has two main effects, the first in causing symptoms of allergy, such as hives, itching, and congestion, and the second in producing stomach acid. (Strictly speaking, it also has a third action, on the brain, but this is not well understood.) Each of these actions relies upon a different type of structure, called a receptor, on the surfaces of cells. The receptor responsible for allergies is designated H_1, and the one responsible for acid production H_2. Thus a histamine$_2$ receptor antagonist would be expected to decrease stomach acid. (The regular kind of antihistamine is just called an antihistamine, not an H_1RA.) In medical literature you will see the term abbreviation H_2RA, but here it will be simplified to HRA.

When HRAs first came out they were available only by prescription and proved invaluable for treating ulcers of the stomach and duodenum (the part of the small intestine adjacent to the stomach), ulcers that are referred to as peptic, meaning related to the digestion. Although HRAs decrease all acid production, they do so more when your stomach is empty, so that acid necessary for digestion is still produced, although to a lesser extent. They are very effective but take about an hour to start working. In OTC doses their effects last from about six to ten hours, which is considerably longer than the longest acting antacids taken under optimal conditions.

Currently available HRAs are **cimetidine, nizatidine, famotidine,** and **ranitidine.** Table 7 attempts to make some sense out of the claims and counterclaims you see in commercials. *Prevention* and *Relief* refer to the symptom of heartburn.

Table 7. Histamine receptor antagonists

Brand Name	Chemical Name	Prevention	Relief	Equivalent dose (mg)
Axid AR	**Nizatidine**	X	(b)	75
Pepcid AC	**Famotidine**	X	X	10
Tagamet HB	**Cimetidine**	X	X	250 (a)
Zantac 75	**Ranitidine**	(b)	X	75

(a) This dose is higher than the FDA approved OTC dose, which is 200 milligrams. It is not known whether this makes much difference as a practical matter.

(b) Although not approved by the FDA for this indication, there is little doubt that medically all of these drugs have equivalent effects.

Although the doses are different, these drugs should be considered to be more or less interchangeable; if your symptoms don't respond to one they are not likely to respond to another. One product claims that it reduces heartburn "completely," but there is no evidence that it is any more complete than any of the others. Some Tagamet commercials point out that it (Tagamet) works faster than Pepcid-AC, which is technically true, but the Pepcid AC lasts longer, and it is doubtful whether this makes much of a difference, since neither of them starts to act in less than an hour and so are not indicated for quick relief.

Cimetidine (Tagamet), however, is slightly different from the others in its effects on the body and in prescription doses, which are higher, has side effects and drug interactions the others do not have. In OTC doses these side effects are minimal. Some doctors, in fact, consider the small OTC doses of all HRAs to be nothing more than expensive antacids.

If your heartburn doesn't respond to antacids or HRAs, see a doctor. Testing and prescription medications may be indicated. You should also seek medical attention if your heartburn is associated with difficulty or pain when swallowing or with intestinal bleeding. Even if they relieve your symptoms adequately, be careful if you find yourself in constant need of them—you may have an ulcer.

Ulcers

No OTC product is labelled for treatment of stomach or duodenal (the portion of the intestine next to the stomach) ulcers because there is no way for you to diagnose them yourself. You certainly may suspect you have one, but that is not the same as knowing for certain. The most accurate diagnostic test is performed with an endoscope, a flexible tube that is passed into the stomach for direct examination.

Pain caused by an ulcer usually occurs about two or two and a half hours after eating or in the middle of the night, and is a steady burning, aching, or gnawing almost in the middle of the upper abdomen. The pain is sometimes described as similar to hunger pangs. It is relieved almost immediately by food or an antacid. The pain is usually not present as one wakes in the morning. This pain, however, is not a constant feature of ulcers, and a good proportion of people with them have no pain at all and only find out after an episode of intestinal bleeding. This is particularly the case when the ulcer is caused by taking too many OTC or prescription internal analgesics such as **aspirin, ibuprofen, ketoprofen,** or **naproxen.**

These medication ulcers, called NSAID induced, are in fact the second most common type, the other being infection with the bacterium called *Helicobacter pylori* (HP).

The interesting thing about HP infection as a cause of ulcers is that when the idea was first proposed the very thought of it was incomprehensible to most doctors. The notion that a germ could survive in the stomach, with its high concentration of hydrochloric acid, seemed ridiculous. What was not realized is how adaptable germs can be. In retrospect, the way HP survives seems simple enough: it manufactures its very own antacid, then flourishes beneath a coating of it.

Although OTC antacids and HRAs will alleviate the symptoms and may even heal an ulcer, the proper treatment nowadays is to eradicate the HP. There are several ways to do this, but all require prescription antibiotics. In addition, the drug Carafate (chemical name sucralfate) may be prescribed. This is neither an antacid nor an HRA, but a substance that coats and protects the ulcer, allowing it to heal. The FDA is considering changing the status of sucralfate to make it available OTC.

Recommendations

If altering your eating habits and the position of your bed don't help your heartburn, try an antacid with a combination of aluminum and **magnesium.** Riopan is a good choice because of its low sodium content but ranks low in taste tests. If you experience diarrhea, switch to an aluminum product. If you become constipated, go to **magnesium.** If you can't tolerate either aluminum or **magnesium,** try products containing **calcium carbonate,** such as Tums or a generic equivalent.

The right dose of an antacid depends on many variables. Follow the instructions and try to use the smallest amount you can. Stop when you feel better. For long term use see a doctor.

Also see a doctor before going to one of the HRAs. This is not because they are unsafe but just to make certain that's what you need.

Remember that there is a high placebo effect with drugs labelled as antacids. Also, the body tends to take care of itself. By the time an antacid starts to work for heartburn, for instance, the acid may have already been partially diluted with your own saliva, which contains bicarbonate, a natural antacid.

As always, make sure you read labels. Alka-Seltzer caplets and gelcaps, for instance, contain **calcium carbonate,** whereas the effervescent tablets contain **sodium bicarbonate.**

17

HEMORRHOIDS AND ANAL PROBLEMS

A hemorrhoid is an enlarged vein. Medically, hemorrhoids can be classified as being internal or external, depending on whether they are inside or outside the opening of the anus. They can also be classified according to how big they are and whether they contain blood clots (thromboses), and whether or not they are prolapsed—extend from inside to outside the anus. In addition, if they are prolapsed, they can be further classified according to whether or not they can be reduced, that is, returned into the rectum.

Unless you're experienced in the matter, you're not likely to be classifying your own hemorrhoids. The symptom you are likely to experience is a lump or sense of fullness in the anal area. The lump may be large or small, soft or firm. There may be tenderness or pain. The pain may feel as if it goes deep inside or may be more superficial. If a blood clot forms, there may be great sensitivity and generally a good deal of discomfort. Although a thrombosed hemorrhoid is usually not dangerous and will usually resolve in a few days, the sudden appearance of a painful lump around the anus is enough to cause many people alarm and will send them to a doctor. Many others, however, will be too embarrassed to seek medical attention.

There are lots of theories about why hemorrhoids form, but one certain cause is increasing pressure within the abdomen. This is why they are so common in pregnancy and in those who sit on the toilet for a long time or who have to strain when having a bowel movement or are chronically constipated.

The available OTC products for hemorrhoid relief and related anal problems usually consist of a combination of ingredients that fall into one of four categories: anesthetics, protectants, decongestants, and astringents.

Anesthetics

Local anesthetics reduce pain by chemically deadening nerve transmissions. They do nothing to alter the disease itself, only the symptoms of the disease. The following anesthetics are available: **benzocaine, benzyl alcohol, dibucaine,** and **pramoxine.**

Although they are all about equally effective, **benzocaine,** present in Americaine Hemorrhoidal Ointment, Lanacane Creme, and Medicone Ointment, has the most potential for causing allergic sensitivity and should be avoided. The others produce irritation much more rarely.

The main difficulty with local anesthetics, however, is not that they may make the problem worse but that their effects only last about an hour. Applying a medication more frequently than this is not recommended.

Astringents

An astringent is a substance that causes contraction of tissues. There are two available, **witch hazel** and **zinc oxide.** Both are ancient remedies that have a long record of safety, although **witch hazel** contains **alcohol,** which can irritate if used too zealously.

Decongestants

Ephedrine and **phenylephrine** are the two decongestants currently available OTC . They are similar and work to reduce swelling by narrowing blood vessels. This effect is different from that of an astringent; decongestants are both stronger and longer lasting. Both are absorbed to some extent through mucous membranes and carry warnings cautioning against use in those with heart disease, high blood pressure, thyroid disease, diabetes, and prostate enlargement. They also should not be used with certain drugs for high blood pressure or depression.

Protectants

As their name implies, protectants are meant to remain on the surface of sensitive tissue to prevent irritation, such as that caused by rubbing. Since they are not absorbed, they have no actual medical effects. The following are available: **cocoa butter, cornstarch** (topical starch), **glycerin, hard fat, kaolin, mineral oil, lanolin, petrolatum** (petroleum jelly), **shark liver oil,** and **zinc oxide.** They are often combined in various proportions and in different concentrations according to a series of complicated formulas developed by the FDA. **Zinc oxide,** for example, which is the main ingredient in calamine lotion, can be classified as either an astringent or as a protectant, depending upon what other ingredients are present.

There is no evidence that one protectant works better than any other or that one combination works better than any other combination. All carry a very low risk of irritation and are very safe. Many of these substances also serve as vehicles or solvents for actual medications in other skin care products.

Available products

The commercial preparations are conglomerations of the above ingredients. The following are examples:

- Anusol suppositories: **cornstarch.**
- Anusol ointment: **pramoxine, mineral oil, zinc oxide.**
- Hemorid Creme and Ointment: **petrolatum, mineral oil, pramoxine, phenylephrine.**
- Hemorid Suppositories: **zinc oxide, phenylephrine, hard fat.**
- Nupercainal Ointment: **dibucaine.**
- Preparation H Ointment: **petrolatum, mineral oil, shark liver oil, phenylephrine.**
- Preparation H Cream: **petrolatum, glycerin, shark liver oil, phenylephrine.**
- Preparation H Suppositories: **cocoa butter, shark liver oil.**
- Tronolane cream: **pramoxine.**

84

- Tronolane suppositories: **zinc oxide, hard fat.**
- Tucks Pads: **witch hazel, glycerin.**
- Tucks Clear Gel: **benzyl alcohol, witch hazel, glycerin.**

Making a selection from these and other available products is not easy, but on the whole, a cream or ointment makes more sense than a suppository. Since the most troublesome symptom is likely to be pain or itching rather than swelling, one of the local anesthetics such as **pramoxine** would probably be best.

Don't use any of these products for more than a week; if your symptoms have not subsided you should definitely see a doctor, as you should if there is any associated rectal bleeding. You should also discontinue use if it seems that the symptoms are getting worse.

Other anal problems

Hemorrhoids are not the only things that can cause masses or growths in the area of the anus and rectum. Boils, warts, and skin tags (areas of excess or redundant skin), are also common. Other diseases, such as anal fissures, anal fistulas, pinworms, or eczema can produce varying degrees of pain, burning, itching, and bleeding.

The anus is an extremely sensitive area even in its healthy state and becomes irritated very easily from toilet paper, feces, undergarments, and sexual contact. Irritation of this kind often causes itching, and itching of the anus deserves special mention.

It is a very common symptom, the medical term for which is pruritus ani. This is Latin for itching of the anus, and is just a fancy way of saying what you already know. Pruritus ani tends to be chronic, and those who suffer from it often go from doctor to doctor in an attempt to find a cure. Most often the condition is a local form of the itch-scratch eczema cycle (Chapter 24, Skin, Hair, and Nails) in which the constant local irritation produces bouts of itching, with resultant scratching and further irritation.

In the long run, however, the condition can become very stubborn, so the earlier it is treated the better. OTC **hydrocortisone** should help, along with strict avoidance of further irritation. As with hemorrhoids, prevention is the best form of treatment.

Recommendations

Use the toilet for bowel movements, not as a library. *Never* bring any reading material into the bathroom with you. Wait until you feel the urge to evacuate, then do it.

Avoid straining. If you are constipated, add fruits, fiber, and fluids to your diet. If that doesn't work, try a bulk-forming laxative. If you have trouble passing hard stool, try the stool softener **docusate.**

After bowel movements wash gently with mild soap and water rather than rubbing with toilet tissue. Toilet tissue should be soft, unscented, and undyed.

Try not to expel flatus (fart) forcefully. When gas escapes in a rush some feces sprays out and is deposited around the opening of the anus. This can cause irritation.

18

MENSTRUAL CRAMPS AND PMS

Cramps

The cramping pain that occurs around the time of menstrual periods in the lower abdomen and back can be very debilitating in some women. It is important to understand that it is a natural function of the uterus: the cramps are related to contractions that help to empty the uterus of the blood and tissue that form menstrual fluid. These cramps are similar to but milder than the cramps that occur during childbirth or miscarriage.

The contractions have been shown to be a result of certain naturally occurring chemicals called prostaglandins. Many, although not all, women who experience severe menstrual cramps also have high levels of prostaglandins. It is for this reason that the newer internal analgesics such as **ibuprofen** (Advil), **ketoprofen** (Orudis KT), and **naproxen** (Aleve) have become so popular for menstrual difficulties—they are good at reducing the synthesis of prostaglandins. These internal analgesics can be considered interchangeable, although there are slight differences in side effects. **Ibuprofen** tends to be tolerated best. For best results, the drugs should be taken to prevent rather than treat the cramps. If you wait for cramps to develop it is usually too late. Take the recommended doses, therefore, for the first two to three days of your period, when prostaglandin synthesis is highest.

A number of combination menstrual products are on the OTC market but are of questionable value. Midol Menstrual Formula, for instance, contains **acetaminophen** (Tylenol), **caffeine**, and **pyrilamine**. The **acetaminophen** is present for its analgesic effect, but you are better off with one of the NSAIDs described above. The **caffeine** is there as a diuretic (to promote water excretion) but in most people it probably doesn't have much of an effect. Furthermore, if you take the maximum dose, which is eight caplets or gelcaps a day, you will be ingesting 480 extra milligrams of **caffeine** per day, the equivalent of about five cups of coffee, and the added jitteriness you are likely to experience will surely counteract any relief of bloating. **Pyrilamine** is an antihistamine, the same type of drug present in most allergy relief products, and whether it helps menstrual cramps is very questionable. It may also cause troublesome sedation. Pamprin Multi-Symptom Formula is similar but substitutes the diuretic **pamabrom** for **caffeine**. **Pamabrom** is actually related to **caffeine** but is not a stimulant and can be purchased separately, if desired.

Younger women, especially teenagers and women in their early twenties suffer most from menstrual cramps. As women get older, especially if they have given birth, the cramping becomes less severe.

PMS

About seventy-five percent of women report some form of discomfort in the week prior to their period, but there is great variation in these symptoms and in their severity. Emotional problems, such as mood swings, hostility, irritability, anxiety, depression, difficulty concentrating, disinterest in work, withdrawal from social situations, and insomnia, may occur, along with headaches, breast pain, fluid retention, bloating, weight gain, and muscle aches and pains. Exactly what is meant by premenstrual syndrome (PMS) is controversial, but several attempts at establishing guidelines for the diagnosis have been published. The American Psychiatric Association, in the Diagnostic and Statistical Manual-IV (DSM), gives criteria for premenstrual dysphoric disorder, an especially severe form of PMS that can actually manifest itself with suicidal thoughts. The diagnosis is based entirely on symptoms, since there are no tests to confirm it, although some studies have shown irregularities of serotonin and **melatonin** secretion in those who suffer extreme forms of PMS.

In the most typical pattern, symptoms are most prominent during the week prior to the onset of menstruation and end in about the middle of the menstrual period. There are usually no symptoms whatever in the week following the period. PMS usually begins in the teenage years or twenties, gets worse with age, and disappears with menopause. It is interesting that most women with PMS do not suffer much from painful periods (dysmenorrhea), and vice versa.

The OTC combinations labelled for PMS relief are often identical to those for regular menstrual discomfort and usually contain **acetaminophen, pamabrom,** and **pyrilamine** (but not **caffeine).** Again, you're better off going with the NSAID analgesics used for menstrual cramps: **ibuprofen, ketoprofen,** or **naproxen.** Anticipating difficulties and taking medications either before or shortly after symptoms develop is most effective.

Nutritional supplements such as **vitamin B6,** calcium, or **magnesium** are sometimes touted for PMS but there is little evidence that they work. Exercise and relaxation techniques, on the other hand, may be very useful.

If your symptoms are debilitating, you may need to see a doctor. Prescription antianxiety or antidepressant medications are effective and may be used in severe cases.

19

MOUTH AND TEETH

Two large organizations act as watchdogs for oral hygiene products, the Food and Drug Administration (FDA) and the American Dental Association (ADA). The ADA studies and evaluates manufacturers' claims and bestows a seal of approval on those that pass muster. It also provides guidelines for the wording on labels and provides information and assistance to the FDA.

Toothpaste

There really is no magic to preventing cavities: regular brushing and flossing are your best weapons. Gimmicks such as Water Piks, ultrasonic cleaners, or electric toothbrushes provide help for the handicapped, but habit and elbow grease are still the best.

Although you will not see it listed as an active ingredient, the basic component of a toothpaste is its abrasive, the general rule being that the milder the abrasive, the better. **Sodium bicarbonate** (baking soda), which is all the rage, is an example of such a mild abrasive and is found in many toothpastes, but it is not superior to others such as **aluminum oxide, aluminum silicate, silica** or **calcium carbonate**. It does, however, raise the pH (reduces the acidity) in the mouth, which is considered to be beneficial to oral tissues. Besides various flavorings and chemicals to make toothpastes foam, the only other important ingredient in a toothpaste is **fluoride**.

Fluoride in some form has been shown convincingly to play an important role in preventing cavities, and many municipal water supplies are fluoridated for this reason. **Fluoride** works best when taken internally, but direct application to the teeth in the form of a toothpaste or mouthwash is also effective.

Fluoride in toothpastes may be delivered by **sodium monofluorophosphate, sodium fluoride,** or **stannous fluoride.** Although they are all probably equally effective, the extra-strength **sodium monofluorophosphate** product (Aim Extra Strength) may be a better cavity fighter than the regular strength variety, but it must be used with particular caution in children.

Kids should be supervised, in fact, whenever they brush their teeth, because they often swallow toothpaste and may ingest too much fluoride. Young children should be taught never to swallow toothpaste or mouthwash.

The labels on some toothpastes promise superiority in fighting plaque or tartar. This can be confusing. Tartar, or calculus, is the end stage of a natural process by which a coat forms on teeth. The first stage of this coating is called pellicle and the second is called plaque. Bacteria collect in the plaque and it thickens. When plaque becomes calcified it is called tartar. The tartar can, in turn, lead to more plaque, first on the teeth above the gum line, then on the teeth below the gum line. At this point it can be removed at home, but once it spreads lower it can lead to gum (periodontal) disease, including bone destruction.

The claim that a toothpaste reduces plaque really doesn't mean too much, because all toothpastes reduce plaque to some extent, as does simple brushing, even without a toothpaste. A new toothpaste, however, Colgate Total, which contains the antibacterial ingredient **triclosan,** slows the formation of plaque by inhibiting the aggregation of bacteria in it. The stabilized form of **stannous fluoride** (in Crest Gum Control), which inhibits the metabolism of bacteria, may work similarly. Both of these toothpastes are approved for prevention of gingivitis (inflammation of the gums).

The tartar control ingredients (**pyrophosphates** and **zinc citrate**) work to prevent *calcification* of the plaque, not its formation, and unfortunately, they only help prevent tartar above the gum line, so real benefits are very questionable.

You may also see special commercial chemical products

that claim to reduce plaque (the second stage) itself. At the present time plaque removal and plaque control systems are still being studied and evaluated by the FDA and ADA, for although there is evidence that some chemical ingredients can indeed reduce plaque, at present no OTC product is approved for that labelling.

Toothbrushes

Most people don't buy a new toothbrush often enough. The general recommendation is that they be replaced every three months or so because of contamination and wear. Most dentists prefer soft bristles, although what soft means can vary from manufacturer to manufacturer. Small heads are also generally preferred, especially for children, although if you have a large mouth and large teeth, a bigger head might be more efficient. Select one with the ADA seal and buy more than one at a time (perhaps when they are on sale) to keep them on hand. How often and how properly you brush is more important than the brand name. Rinse thoroughly after each use.

Electric toothbrushes are available for those who have handicaps such as arthritis, nerve damage, or muscle disease. Ultrasonsic cleaners do a similar job but are more expensive.

Dental floss

The purpose of dental floss is to remove plaque and food particles from places you can't reach with your toothbrush. As with toothbrushes, it doesn't much matter which type you use, waxed, unwaxed, thin, thick, or low-friction fiber. If the spaces between your teeth are close together, however, you might try one of the low-friction types, such as Glide, or one of the threader devices that help insert the floss between your teeth. Similarly, if you are handicapped or not particularly dextrous, one of the flossing aids might be useful. Although you should floss once a day, treating all tooth spaces, don't be too vigorous near your gums because they are easy to injure. Choose a floss with the ADA seal of approval and buy the economy size.

Toothpicks are another way of cleaning between the teeth, but they can't reach as far as floss. Round, flat, and soft triangular types, such as Stim-U-Dent, are available. Tiny brushes, such as the Proxabrush, are similar, but should not substitute for flossing. The soft rubber tips on some toothbrush handles, however, may provide an added beneficial effect when used to gently massage the gums.

You can test your cleaning technique every so often with an OTC disclosing agent, which is a vegetable dye that stains plaque. These are available either as solutions or as chewable tablets. To use them follow the manufacturer's directions.

Water piks and other water irrigation systems

These are not substitutes for brushing and flossing, but can help remove food from hard to reach areas. There are two types, pulsating and steady stream. Neither has been shown to be superior, but the steady-stream types are cheaper. As a rule, do not use either of them at a higher setting than medium.

Tooth whitenening

The early 1990s saw a big brouhaha among manufacturers, the American Dental Association, and the FDA over the subject of tooth whiteners. The manufacturers wanted more freedom to market these lucrative products, the FDA wanted more control, and the ADA took a stand somewhere in the middle.

Part of the problem is a controversy regarding the role of peroxide.

Originally, a dentist named Keyes advised his patients with gum disease to mix **hydrogen peroxide** (peroxide) and **sodium bicarbonate** (baking soda) together and to brush their teeth with the resulting sludge. It sounded good; it was cheap and natural, and soon other dentists began making the same recommendation. But dentists were also using peroxide as a bleach, and soon commercial OTC products were being developed and sold as tooth whiteners.

Because of concerns about the peroxide, the FDA issued warning letters to the manufacturers, claiming that tooth whitening was not cosmetic but rather a form of drug therapy. The companies retaliated with a coalition disputing this opinion, and then the ADA got into the fray, coming down on the side of the FDA. Lawsuits were threatened. At present there are a number of whitening toothpastes, some of which contain **hydrogen peroxide** or potent abrasives. The Natural White and Pearl Drops product lines, however, contain **titanium dioxide,** a white pigment that produces temporary whitening but does not bleach.

The issue revolves around the safety of peroxide, including **carbamide peroxide,** which is contained in products marketed to dentists for home use by their patients. Indeed, there are some doctors and dentists who do not believe peroxide products have any place in medicine because of the damage they do to tissues, but the truth is probably somewhere in between.

Until more data are available, if you want your teeth whitened or bleached, have it done under your dentist's care. Peroxides do irritate oral tissues and highly abrasive toothpastes can cause tooth damage by removing enamel.

Denture cleansers

Denture cleansers come in two forms: those for brushing and those for soaking. Good denture care requires both types of cleaning.

Those for brushing are like toothpastes and are formulated from the same ingredients as regular toothpastes, such as **calcium carbonate** and **silica,** but are milder. It is best not to use regular toothpastes on dentures because they are generally more harsh.

The cleansers designed for soaking come as tablets or powders and are designed to be dissolved in water. There are several types of these that contain multiple ingredients, such as the Efferdent and Polident product lines, but most rely upon the release of **hydrogen peroxide** in an alkaline solution to do the job. Look for the ADA seal of approval and follow manufacturer's directions carefully.

Calcified coatings on your dentures can be loosened by soaking them for ten or fifteen minutes in a solution of one part white household vinegar to nine parts water. Always rinse your dentures thoroughly after cleaning and before putting them back into your mouth.

Denture adhesives

The simple fact about denture adhesives is this: If your denture is fitting properly you shouldn't need them. Wear and tear and the loss of the bony structure of your mouth mean that dentures require periodic readjustement. Frequent use of adhesives can actually cause increased bone loss by aggravating the misalignment between your dentures and gums. Furthermore, adhesives should never be used where there is mixed dentition (in which some natural teeth remain) because their acidity can remove calcium from the natural teeth. On the other hand, some people like the feeling of confidence they get from denture adhesives. As long as your dentures fit properly, minimal amounts of adhesive are probably safe.

Bad breath

Most people suffer from bad breath (also known as oral malodor or halitosis) occasionally. It clearly has a strong psychological component. One study found that people, particularly if they are sensitive to their relationship with others or obsessive-compulsive, tend to overestimate the foulness of their breaths. This study actually employed a person to act as judge, into whose face the test subjects breathed. The subjects usually thought that their breath was worse than it really was. On the other hand, it is possible to be oblivious to the problem. The FDA says: "Unless a social contact informs an individual that he or she has malodor, the individual may be unaware of its presence." So you have to be aware of your own insecurities in the matter, and possibly, although this is tricky, rely upon the honesty of your intimate contacts.

Bad breath can come from medical conditions such as liver disease, kidney disease, diabetes, tooth decay, and certain infections, but the common forms of it occur for one of three reasons, smoking, eating smelly foods, or having germs in the mouth.

The solution to the bad breath from smoking is to stop smoking.

The foods that are most often associated with mouth odor are garlic and onions, which, if they weren't so plentiful, would be considered great delicacies. Garlic and onions contain oils that are not digested but rather recirculate in the saliva, producing prolonged bad breath. Toothpastes, mouthwashes, mints, lozenges, or Breath Assure can be used to cover up these odors, to a point.

The persistent bad breath caused by bacterial overgrowth, however, is not easily treated. Some individuals just seem to support the growth of these germs more than other individuals. Bacteria tend to grow on the back of the tongue in a thick coating. Antibacterial solutions or mouthwashes can help, but actual physical removal of the coating is needed. To keep the odor from returning you have to continue to do this; removing the coat just once isn't enough. You can try a toothbrush or use one of the special scrapers designed for the purpose. A dentist can diagnose the condition and show you how to perform the procedure. Using a homemade mouthwash may also be helpful. Try rinsing with a solution of one teaspoonful of **sodium bicarbonate** (baking soda) in a half glass of water.

Mouthwashes

The status of mouthwashes, which are also called mouthrinses, is controversial. This is mainly because most of them contain **alcohol,** which may contribute to oral cancer, particularly in tobacco users. Since these cancers may take decades to develop adequate studies are difficult to perform. Those who want to be safe should not use a mouthwash with **alcohol.**

Several mouthwashes, such as Listerine, (which is 26.9 percent **alcohol)** have approved wording on their labels that says they help to "prevent and reduce" plaque. Although there is scientific evidence for this claim, exactly how much it helps is not known, and it may be found that, on balance, long term use does more harm than good. Besides **alcohol,** Listerine contains **eucalyptol, thymol, methyl salicylate,** and **menthol,** the combination of which also has antiseptic qualities. Other mouthwashes contain antiseptics such as **cetylpyridinium chloride** to provide their beneficial effects. It should be noted, however, that antiseptics are indiscriminate in their action and also kill friendly bacteria.

Some mouthwashes use a detergent, such as **sodium lauryl sulfate** (also used to foam toothpastes), to fight plaque before brushing. One example of such a product is Advanced Formula Plax. The detergent is said to help loosen the plaque and makes it easier to remove, but the effectiveness of this is controversial.

Most people use mouthwashes for bad breath, and for this purpose very occasional use is probably not dangerous. Personal preferences would dictate the choice of a green mint, blue mint, red cinammon, or a medicinal flavor.

Mouthwashes or rinses which contain **sodium fluoride** are a different matter and have been shown to reduce cavities. They are particularly useful if you wear braces or live in an area where drinking water is not fluoridated.

Canker sores

Canker sores (aphthous ulcers or aphthae) are very common. No one knows what causes them, although they are almost certainly caused by an infection (or a reaction to an infection) of some kind. The type of infection is not known but it is not herpes. The sores are usually found on the palate, cheeks, or gums and are very painful and very sensitive. They may be small or large and appear sharply defined (punched out), with a white center and a red border. Unlike an injury, such as biting the inside of your lip or cheek, a canker sore usually persists longer, for about five to seven days. Unfortunately, many may develop in succession, causing continuous and considerable discomfort.

Of the numerous available OTC products, none shortens the duration of the problem or works very well. FDA approved anesthetics include **benzocaine, benzyl alcohol, camphor, dyclonine, lidocaine, menthol,** and **phenol,** but these are good only for very temporary relief (up to an hour). Most commercial products contain **benzocaine,** either alone or in combination with other ingredients. Plain Orabase (there are other products in the Orabase line) is a simple non-medicated protective coating that, although not an anesthetic, may provide some relief. As an alternative, **benzoin** can be used the same way. The problem with applying things to oral mucous membranes is that they wash away quickly.

A still different approach to treating canker sores is to use a wound cleanser. There are two of these, **hydrogen perox-**

ide, such as Peroxyl Oral Spot Treatment, and **carbamide peroxide,** such as Gly-Oxide or Orajel Perioseptic. These are of very questionable value, however, and usually sting quite a bit when applied.

Although not approved by the FDA as an OTC canker sore reliever, the antihistamine **diphenhydramine** (Benadryl) has some local anesthetic properties. Liquid forms of it can be swished around inside of the mouth for one minute three times a day and then spit out. Make sure it is plain and pure **diphenhydramine;** many cough and cold preparations contain multiple ingredients. One way to make the **diphenhydramine** stick better is to mix it with **magnesium hydroxide** suspension (milk of magnesia), half and half. Again, make sure you do not swallow the mixture.

Not all oral ulcers are canker sores, and it may be wise, if you aren't sure about what's going on, to have the diagnosis confirmed by a doctor. A prescription medication, Aphthasol paste (amlexanox), has been shown to shorten the duration of the ulcers by about a day and a half.

Chapped lips

Dry, cracked, swollen, and burning lips (cheilitis) most often occurs in the winter as a result of dry, cold air. The problem is almost always aggravated by lip licking. Although the evaporation of saliva feels nice and cool to hot lips, the saliva eventually causes even more drying. Saliva also contains enzymes, and when it is comes in contact with the lips it partially digests them.

Step one, therefore, in combatting chapped lips, is to stop licking.

Step two is to apply an occlusive barrier. Theoretically any moisturizer might do, but practically speaking a heavy product like **petrolatum** (petroleum jelly) is best. The lipstick-like applicators are convenient and popular.

If that doesn't work, use a **hydrocortisone** ointment (not the cream) three or four times a day for a week or two. If that doesn't help, you'll need a doctor. What looks like chapping, particularly on the lower lip, year round may be a precancerous condition from sun exposure.

Cold sores

Cold sores, also called fever blisters, are caused by a herpes virus that is almost exactly the same as the one implicated in genital herpes. This virus is unique in that the infection actually lasts a lifetime but symptoms only occur (recur) at intervals, every few weeks to every few years, because the virus actually exists in a dormant form within the cutaneous nerves. Something, such as sunlight, another viral illness such as a cold or intestinal infection, or physical stress, triggers the virus to come out of its inactive state.

The usual pattern includes an initial period of sensitivity, tingling, burning, or swelling, followed by a crop of tiny blisters in a cluster. The blisters dry up into a scab and the scab falls off. The whole process takes a week or two to run its course.

There is nothing you can buy on your own to shorten the course of a cold sore; the most you can hope for is some decrease in the pain and discomfort. Oral drugs such as lysine, pyridoxine (**vitamin B₆**), or lactobacillus, are worthless.

Some preparations labelled for cold sores are actually sunscreens in lip balm form. It is a good idea to protect your lips carefully from the sun to prevent an outbreak of cold sores, but applying the sunscreen after a sore appears is too late.

Although the FDA has categorized a number of ingredients as safe and effective for herpes, it should be remembered that they are only for symptomatic relief. As with canker sores, most of the available products contain **benzocaine** with other ingredients (counterirritants) such as **menthol, camphor,** or **phenol.** The problem with **benzocaine** is that some people are allergic to it and can develop quite a severe reaction. This can be avoided by using **lidocaine** containing products. Allergic reactions to **lidocaine** are very uncommon.

Keeping the area moist with plain **petrolatum** applied several times a day is probably as good a treatment as any of the others. There are prescription drugs such as famcyclovir (Famvir), acyclovir (Zovirax), or valcyclovir (Valtrex), which, if taken early in an attack, will abort it, and if taken constantly will prevent all future attacks.

There is another condition—called perlèche, or angular stomatitis—that deserves to be mentioned because it is sometimes confused with herpes. This shows up as a crack or split in one or both corners of the mouth and is mainly due to irritation from saliva in those who wear dentures or braces and who constantly lick the corners of their mouths. Once the irritation begins a yeast *(Candida)* infection may develop and lead to a chronic problem. Treatment is to avoid licking and to apply a mixture of 1 percent **hydrocortisone** cream and either **clotrimazole** cream or **miconazole** cream two or three times a day for about a week.

Dry mouth

An excessively dry mouth can be the result of anxiety, medications (such as antihistamines and antihypertensives), diseases of the glands that produce saliva, autoimmune diseases (such as Sjögren's syndrome), aging, or mouth-breathing from nasal obstruction. Candies or lozenges may help, but their sugar content is a definite disadvantage. Artificial salivas usually employ **cellulose ethers,** similar to those in artificial tears, to mimic natural saliva. They are available as liquids, sprays, and swabs.

Sensitive teeth

A sensitive tooth can signify the onset of an abscess or of periodontal problems, so don't treat yourself with a sensitive-tooth product without a diagnosis from a dentist. The usual cause of sensitive teeth is exposure of portions of the roots of the teeth from gum disease, braces, injury, oral surgery, or excessive brushing or flossing. Scrubbing across the gumline can cause sensitivity by producing abrasions at the neck of the teeth.

If your dentist recommends a desensitizer, the only approved ingredient is **potassium nitrate,** which is found in a number of products. It can take up to two weeks to work and is not recommended in children under twelve. To further take care of sensitive teeth use a low abrasive toothpaste and avoid those labelled for tooth whitening.

Teething

It is a well known fact that babies whose teeth are coming in cry a lot. It is also a well known fact that babies whose teeth are *not* coming in cry a lot. It is always risky for adults to diagnose the ills of children who cannot pinpoint the source of their discomfort. In this case the crying may very well have nothing whatever to do with teething. It is interesting that children whose teeth are coming in for the second time, that is, who are getting their permanent teeth, don't seem to cry as much. If your pediatrician believes that your child's teething is causing discomfort, however, there are several products containing **benzocaine** available, such as Baby Orajel Teething Pain Medicine and Orabase Baby Analgesic Teething Gel. In any event, it is important to note that teething does not cause fever, a runny nose, chest congestion, enlarged glands, vomiting, or diarrhea. If any of these symptoms is present the problem is not teething.

20

NAUSEA AND VOMITING

Although nausea is generally defined as the sensation that preceeds vomiting, and although one can experience nausea without vomiting, the two symptoms are best considered together.

There are many causes of nausea and vomiting. These causes range from things as minor as being emotionally upset to things as serious as having a brain tumor. Intestinal flu, food poisoning, pregnancy, motion sickness, appendicitis, liver disease, kidney disease, diseases of the ear, heart attacks, and chemotherapy may all be accompanied by prominent nausea and vomiting.

In some cases, as in poisoning, vomiting is clearly a protective mechanism designed to rid the body of noxious substances, but in most other situations its biological function is not well understood.

Nausea itself is not dangerous, but vomiting can be. In someone with disease or weakness of the blood vessels of the stomach or esophagus, one episode of forceful vomiting may cause serious hemorrhage. Prolonged vomiting can result in loss of fluid, electrolytes (charged ions in the blood), and stomach acid, which can cause both dehydration and the condition known as alkalosis, in which the natural acid-base balance of the blood is disrupted. This can be particularly serious in children, especially since diarrhea may also be present. One major problem in treating prolonged vomiting is that when you can't keep anything down oral medications are useless.

For the most part, the OTC nausea medications are most useful in treating motion sickness.

Motion sickness is caused by confusion in your brain between what your eyes are telling you and what your inner ears (labyrinths) are telling you. Children seem to experience it the most, especially in cars, but if things get bad enough just about anyone will succumb, particularly on boats and ships in rough waters. It's helpful to anticipate motion sickness, and prevent it if you can; once it starts it is usually too late to treat it effectively.

The approved OTC drugs for motion sickness are all antihistamines: **cyclizine, dimenhydrinate, diphenhydramine,** and **meclizine.** All should be taken at least thirty minutes before the onset of motion, except for **meclizine** (Bonine, Dramamine II), the one most commonly given out free on cruise ships, which should be taken an hour or two before the anticipated roughness. **Meclizine** is the best choice because it is the longest acting. Some people, in fact, find that taking it the night before a boating expedition is helpful, with the effects lasting throughout the next day. The main side effects of all are the same: drowsiness, fatigue, and dry mouth. Drug interactions and precautions are also just about the same for all, but each has a different dose and different recommendations for use in children.

Wristbands, which are also sold on cruise ships, allegedly work by acupressure. These are safe but seem to work best in those who also believe in the Tooth Fairy.

There are other products available for nausea but they have different indications. **Phosphorylated carbohydrate solution,** marketed under several brand names (Cola Syrup, Emetrol, and Especol), are labelled for control of nausea and vomiting and upset stomach caused by viral infections (intestinal flu), overeating, and emotional upset. Some of these products contain lots of sugar and should not be used if you have diabetes. They are designed to be taken every fifteen minutes, which is difficult if you are vomiting frequently. Their effectiveness is questionable.

Bismuth subsalicylate (Pepto-Bismol) is labelled for control of a variety of intestinal complaints, including "indigestion, heartburn, nausea and fullness caused by overindulgence." It is discussed in Chapter 9 on diarrhea.

Morning sickness is another kind of nausea and vomiting, one of the most common symptoms of pregnancy. It is probably caused by the change in hormones and its treatment is very controversial. Even medications that used to be in common use and were thought to be safe have been abandoned as potentially too dangerous. One substance, however, **vitamin B$_6$** (pyridoxine), may have promise. Studies show conflicting results but at least one has shown that twenty-five milligrams every eight hours relieves morning sickness. Still, it is better not to treat yourself for morning sickness; always check with your doctor.

21

NUTRITIONAL SUPPLEMENTS

You had probably learned all you need to know about basic nutrition by the time you were in the third grade and certainly by the sixth. And if you weren't paying attention in school, your mother filled in the blanks. Whether you now act on this knowledge, of course, is a different matter. All of us realize and understand the dangers of a high-fat high-cholesterol diet, and yet there are still many of us who choose to eat a double bacon cheeseburger and fries at every opportunity. However, the knowledge about nutrition is there, and even if you've forgotten it you can easily refresh your memory from a number of reliable sources.

These sources will usually provide you with a simple table of recommended daily allowances (RDAs) of various nutrients. These figures are the result of a series of observations and experiments of animals and humans that have been going on for over a hundred years. In these experiments, test subjects are given diets deficient in one or more substances. The effects of these deficiencies are observed and recorded. Then the substances are replaced and the minimum amount needed to reverse the symptom of deficiency is noted. This isn't the figure you see listed in the tables, though, because it is recognized that people differ somewhat (but not a lot) in their requirements. The figure is larger than the minimum amount to give us some leeway.

Human beings have proved themselves to be adaptable to a wide range of cultural, climactic, and culinary variations. The original Eskimos subsisted quite nicely on a high-fat, high-protein diet of whale blubber, whereas rice farmers in the Mekong Delta of Vietnam rarely taste meat of any kind. The body has a mechanism for dealing with overabundance and scarcity of foods. The general system is called homeostasis: the tendency toward stability.

The world seems divided into those who believe in vitamins and those who don't, as if it were a matter of faith rather than science. The fact of the matter is that the diet of most Americans is sufficient. We do not need supplemental vitamins and minerals; most of us are actually over nourished. Thus, when Americans spend billions of dollars a year on nutritional supplements, most of it is wasted. The reason it is wasted is that the people who tend to buy the stuff don't need it; those who do need it stay malnourished.

The reasons for malnutrition include poverty, alcoholism, psychological disorders, fad diets, intestinal diseases, and the use of certain drugs (which either depress the appetite or interfere with the absorption of nutrients). Some elderly people get into trouble with a diet of tea and toast, which is just another way of saying bread and water. In most cases, deficiencies tend to be multiple rather than single, and the consequence is a symptom or number of symptoms, most of which are hard to diagnose yourself.

There is a certain danger in assuming that because you have a certain symptom there is a vitamin deficiency causing it. The disease known as perlèche, for example, in which the corners of the mouth become red and cracked, is almost always due simply to irritation from saliva, usually from licking. But because a similar symptom can occur in niacin and B vitamin deficiency—along with far more serious things—some people take huge doses of B vitamins to correct the problem. Unfortunately, niacin and the B vitamins can cause significant side effects when taken in large amounts. Similarly, it is known from experimentation on human subjects that one of the side effects of pantothenic acid deficiency is burning and tingling of the feet. But this is in experimental subjects only; isolated pantothenic acid deficiency is extremely rare. The symptom of burning and tingling of the feet is almost never caused by a vitamin deficiency and requires a medical evaluation and work-up.

The most important thing to remember about vitamins is that you need very tiny amounts of them. This is borne out by the fact that most multivitamin pills contain one hundred percent of the RDA of every vitamin and most minerals you need every day.

Information about the various diseases caused by deficiencies of vitamins and minerals can be found in the ingredients section of this book, along with daily requirements and sources of each nutrient.

The following are covered: **niacin, pantothenic acid, the vitamins A, B$_1$, B$_2$, B$_6$, B$_{12}$, C, D, E, K, biotin, carnitine, chromium, copper, magnesium, manganese, molybdenum, phosphorus, selenium, and zinc.** The RDAs are usually given as milligrams (mg) or micrograms (mcg) but sometimes as international units (IU). International units are appropriate when several chemical compounds may be sources for an active nutrient and each compound possesses a different level of activity. Also listed are possible side effects from ingesting too much of a vitamin or mineral.

There are two minerals, however, iron and calcium, and one supplement, **DHEA,** that deserve special attention.

Iron

Iron is important to many body functions and is crucial for the transport of oxygen in red blood cells. Iron deficiency is the most common nutritional deficiency in the United States. Symptoms are variable. Usually by the time they have developed, iron in the body has already been depleted substantially. The classic symptom of iron deficiency is an anemia, which causes weakness, fatigue, shortness of breath, and pallor (paleness). Other symptoms are hair loss and cold extremities. Iron deficiency is much more common in women than in men because of menstruation, and often because of a lower overall dietary iron intake.

Good sources of iron are in liver, red meat, dark green vegetables, egg yolk, dried fruits, beans, peas, potatoes, and grains. Cooking in a cast-iron pot adds iron to your food.

The decreased consumption of red meats in the United States may be good for the health of the nation on balance, but it has increased the incidence of iron deficiency. Although there are other ways to get iron, red meat is the best, since there is a lot of iron in it and it is well absorbed. That's one of the main problems with iron: on average only about ten percent of the amount you eat (or five percent from vegetable sources) makes it into your bloodstream, but the amount absorbed from meat is about twenty percent.

It is also possible to become iron deficient through slow, chronic bleeding, as from an ulcer or intestinal cancer. There are many cases where the first symptom of such hemorrhage was fainting because of anemia. Thus, if you have iron deficiency it is very important to find the cause of it, and for this you need a doctor.

If your doctor decides you need more iron than your diet can provide, the best way to get it is with **ferrous sulfate.** Other forms, such as **ferrous fumarate** or **ferrous gluconate** offer no advantage, although the fumarate contains some-what more iron than the sulfate (thirty-three percent versus twenty percent). All forms of iron can cause upset stomach and constipation. Taking the iron with food will help the upset stomach but will also decrease the amount of iron absorbed. The absorption can be increased, however, by taking it along with **vitamin C.** To avoid constipation you should increase your intake of fruits, vegetables, and liquids. If that doesn't work, the stool softener **docusate** or one of the bulk-forming laxatives might help. (See Chapter 7 for more on this subject.)

Calcium

Calcium is crucial to metabolism and is the major component of bone, each of us containing several pounds of it in our skeletons. Its blood level must be kept within strict limits by the body because either high or low levels can lead to irregularities of the heartbeat (arrhythmias), blood clotting diseases, diseases of the endocrine glands, and diseases of bones. Some of these situations can be critical and can lead to coma and death.

Deficiency of calcium leads to poor bone growth in children and thinning of the bones (osteoporosis) in adults, although the major reason for osteoporosis in women after menopause is decreased estrogen.

Calcium deficiency may be caused by a poor diet or by intestinal diseases (malabsorption), kidney disease, parathyroid disease, vitamin D deficiency, and some drugs, such as anticonvulsants, steroids, and insulin. Prolonged used of aluminum-containing antacids can also lead to low calcium.

A diet adequate in milk and dairy products, dark green leafy vegetables, citrus fruits, beans, and peas should provide enough calcium for most people. Sardines and nonfat yogurt are also good low calorie sources of it. The current RDAs are 600 mg for infants, 800 mg for children under four years, 1000 mg for children over four years and adults, 1200 mg for pregnant and nursing women, and 1200 to 1500 mg for menopausal women. Many calcium supplements are available in a wide array of tablets, capsules, and liquids. These fall into two categories, insoluble, and soluble. The *insoluble* forms, **calcium carbonate** and **calcium phosphate,** contain more calcium but need acidity for absorption and should be taken with meals. The soluble forms, **calcium citrate, calcium lactate,** and **calcium gluconate,** have less calcium but are absorbed better. The soluble preparations are preferred if you are taking a prescription or OTC drug that reduces stomach acid, such as **nizatidine** (Axid AR), **famotidine** (Pepcid AC), **cimetidine** (Tagamet HB), or **ranitidine** (Zantac 75). On the other hand, if you are in need of both an antacid and calcium supplements, you might as well take one of the **calcium carbonate** products for both indications. The generic forms of **calcium carbonate** are very economical.

Too much calcium, however, is also not good for you. Side effects include loss of appetite, nausea, vomiting, and constipation. The most serious problem is the development of kidney stones, which can lead to kidney damage. Taking in large amounts of **vitamin D** will aggravate any disease caused by excess calcium.

DHEA

DHEA (dehydroepiandosterone) is classified as a food supplement, but it is really is nothing of the kind. It's only on the market because of a loophole in the law. The FDA originally banned this product but manufacturers were able to sneak it back in after the Dietary Supplement Health and Education Act of 1994. It is a hormone produced in the adrenal glands of monkeys, humans, and a few other animals.

DHEA is actually a very interesting substance and is the most abundant steroid hormone in the body. It is generally classified as an androgen, or male type hormone, but it is a weak androgen. Even though it is a steroid, it seems to have little specific activity. Rather, it is converted to other hormones, including testosterone and estrogen, within the tissues themselves. Thus, men and women process and metabolize the hormone in different ways. In men, in fact, it may be possible that **DHEA** is converted to estrogen in some tissues, such as the heart, and may thereby prevent heart disease.

In primates **DHEA** is present in very high levels in the fetus, then drops dramatically at birth. It rises again in puberty and young adulthood, then progressively decreases with age. This pattern has given rise to the idea that it might counteract the ageing process.

One study did show a decrease in depression in elderly individuals, along with improved memory. In addition, some preliminary results have shown positive effects on the immune system and cardiovascular system. It might also be helpful in diabetes and autoimmune diseases (in which the immune system reacts against the body's own tissues).

At present, however, there are still far too many unknowns about **DHEA** to recommend it. Hepatitis (inflammation of the liver) and an increase in ovarian cancer are two possible side effects that have already been reported. Others will probably come to the fore as more individuals take **DHEA**.

Some doctors, however, are prescribing it for their patients or are willing to monitor the situation in those who want to try it. If you do want to be a guinea pig, have a **DHEA** blood level, along with other laboratory tests, and a physical exam. Have the tests and the physical exam repeated at scheduled intervals. But don't even consider taking **DHEA** if you are under fifty.

Recommendations

Shop as much as you want in health food stores but don't believe anything the clerk tells you—except for the price of an item. Do your own research before you shop.

The secret to good nutrition is a balanced and diversified diet. It's true that we often don't eat what's good for us. Broccoli, for instance, is a very good food—low in calories and pesticides, high in vitamins and minerals—but many people hate it. If you can't dress up a particular food to make it palatable, something with similar nutritional value can be substituted. In addition, many supermarkets are handing out recipe and nutrition cards in their produce departments to help make eating good foods more enjoyable.

Pregnant women, nursing women, growing children, smokers, those who take birth control pills, heavy drinkers, and strict vegetarians should take one multivitamin a day. Generic products are equivalent to the higher priced name brands. Comparison shop and read the labels—some products offer a greater percentage of the RDAs for each vitamin or mineral than other products.

If you have liver disease, kidney disease, or intestinal disease follow your doctor's advice about supplements.

Don't take supplemental iron unless your doctor has recommended it or unless you have been diagnosed with iron deficiency. There are many causes for fatigue and lack of energy that have nothing to do with iron.

22

PAIN

Pain is both a simple and a complex subject, simple because we all experience it to various degrees, complex because the reasons for it are so numerous and its relief at times so difficult. Chest pain can be due to a muscle strain, pneumonia, or a heart attack; a headache might be due to tension, an impending stroke, or a brain tumor. Books are written about pain, specialists devote themselves to the study of it, and clinics exist solely to treat intractable forms of it. More money is spent on internal pain relievers than any other OTC drug class. To further complicate matters, it is well known that pain thresholds and perceptions differ greatly from person to person, as does the response to analgesic medications.

Before discussing the available products, here are a few words of general advice about pain:

- Don't treat abdominal pain (except menstrual cramps) with internal analgesics. Serious diseases such as ulcers, gall bladder disease, diverticulitis, pancreatitis, peritonitis, or appendicitis may be the underlying cause.
- For a toothache, see a dentist. You may have an abscess. OTC pain relievers can be used *after* the root canal.
- Boils or abscesses, although tending to resolve spontaneously with time, often need drainage or internal antibiotics. Analgesics are rarely enough.
- Headaches, particularly those around the fore-

head, may be due to a sinus infection (sinusitis). These should be treated by a physician.

- OTC pain relievers should be used only for temporary or mild pain. If you have arthritis, you should follow your doctor's recommendations.
- Take the smallest dose you can get by with and go up from there. Doctors who deal with pain will often push analgesics to tolerance (or toxicity), but you can get into trouble—with internal bleeding for example—if you try this yourself. More people die each year from the side effects of OTC analgesics than from skin cancer.
- Remember that pain is a symptom of disease. If you find yourself popping pills continuously because the pain is severe or of unusual character or intensity, see a doctor.
- If you are allergic to one pain reliever described in this chapter, you may be allergic to all of them. Be particularly careful if you have asthma and nasal polyps.

Internal analgesics

Although you will find many products on the shelves, there are basically only five active ingredients to consider: **aspirin, acetaminophen, ibuprofen, ketoprofen,** and **naproxen.** The last three, furthermore, are all in the same general class of drugs called NSAIDs—non-steroidal anti-inflammatory drugs—and are very similar in their actions. Because the main side effects of many of the drugs are abdominal complaints, such as nausea, pain, cramping, heartburn, constipation, diarrhea, gas, and vomiting, which may occur alone or in combination, it is common for physicians and pharmacists to lump these symptoms collectively—and a little pedantically—under the heading of dyspepsia. These symptoms will be indicated here by the term upset stomach.

Aspirin and other salicylates

Aspirin is the oldest analgesic and therefore the one about which we know the most. For years it was the only one available. The old saying, "Take two aspirin and call me in the morning," is an indication of the cavalier way in which aspirin was and is prescribed. Aspirin, however, is actually quite a potent and important drug.

Its main advantage is that it is widely available, relatively safe, and very inexpensive. Its main disadvantage is as a cause of upset stomach, which it tends to do more than do other internal analgesics.

To counteract this, **aspirin** should be taken with foods or lots of water. In addition, there are two techniques drug companies use to soften the blow: buffering and enteric coating.

Buffering refers to the process of adding a small amount of antacid to the preparation. Although this has the effect of reducing stomach acid to a degree, buffering makes **aspirin** more tolerable mainly by speeding its absorption. Bufferin and Ascriptin are the best known of these products, and generics are available.

A special and more potent type of buffering is found in Alka-Seltzer and similar products. In this case, **sodium bicarbonate** (baking soda), a powerful antacid, is used. This reduces stomach acid considerably and greatly speeds the rate of **aspirin** absorption, making these products the fastest acting aspirin pain relievers. Unfortunately, if used chronically, they will also cause your urine to become more alkaline. This will increase the excretion of salicylate—the active component of **aspirin**—in your blood and reduce its beneficial effects. These products also contain very large amounts of sodium, which should be avoided if you are on a sodium restricted diet.

Enteric coating surrounds the **aspirin** pellet with a substance that makes it resistant to stomach acid, delaying digestion until it reaches the small intestine, where the acidity is lower. Unlike buffering, which speeds absorption, enteric coating slows absorption and makes it more difficult to predict when these products will begin to work. Ecotrin is an example of this type of product. Enteric coating is more effective than buffering in reducing irritation to the stomach lining and is most useful in those who are being treated constantly with high doses of aspirin.

A different strategy to avoid upset stomach is to bypass the upper intestinal tract entirely by employing rectal suppositories. Although this works, it is at the expense of delayed, erratic absorption of the drug and can cause a sore anus.

Aspirin continues to be widely used for pain, despite the introduction of newer analgesics. This is partly because of **aspirin**'s effect as a blood thinner. Anticoagulation is real and lasts about a week after taking even a small amount of **aspirin**. A small dose, in fact, may be more effective than a large dose. **Aspirin** has been shown to help prevent blood clots, which may lead to heart attacks and some strokes, and many doctors recommend such treatment prophylactically. There is also evidence to support the use of **aspirin** given as emergency treatment for heart attacks and strokes. One important point to remember, however, is that some strokes are due to cerebral hemorrhage, not blood clots, and if this is the case, **aspirin** will aggravate the situation.

Aspirin is the best known and most potent member of the drug class known as salicylates, all of which possess some pain relieving qualities. There are three other salicylate analgesics available OTC: **magnesium salicylate, sodium salicylate,** and **choline salicylate.**

Magnesium salicylate is found in the Doan's product line and generic drugs that are usually labelled, "for backache." There is nothing whatsoever specific about this drug for backache. Moreover, if your backache is due to kidney disease, the extra magnesium can give you trouble. Although it may cause less of an upset stomach than **aspirin**, **magnesium salicylate** has little to recommend it.

Sodium salicylate is found only in a few combination products and is slightly less effective than **aspirin**. It may be slightly better tolerated, however, in those allergic to **aspirin**.

Choline salicylate is found in one commercial product, Arthropan, as a liquid. It is also less effective than **aspirin** but is absorbed quickly from the stomach.

Similarly, **salicylamide** (which is technically not a salicylate), found in a few combination products, has very little analgesic potency, if any.

No salicylate, including **bismuth subsalicylate** (Pepto-Bismal), should ever be given to children or teenagers fifteen years of age or younger who have symptoms of the flu or chickenpox because they may precipitate the serious disease known as Reye's Syndrome.

Acetaminophen

The best known product containing **acetaminophen** is Tylenol. **Acetaminophen** is very popular for a number of reasons. It is about as effective as **aspirin** for pain but is much better tolerated. It also does not thin (anticoagulate) the blood, making it more suitable for post surgical pain. It is also much safer than **aspirin** in children. Indeed, children under the age of six seem to be particularly resistant to liver damage from overdoses, a protection that adults do not have. It also reduces fever.

Were it not for two other features, **acetaminophen** might be the perfect OTC pain reliever. The first disadvantage is that it is relatively ineffective for menstrual cramps and the second is that it does not reduce inflammation.

The term inflammation can be a difficult concept to grasp. Its classic symptoms are redness, swelling, pain, and reduced function. It is actually a sign of the immune system at work: in a typical infection, for instance, inflammation produces an environment that is hostile to the invading organism. But in other cases, most notably rheumatoid arthritis, inflammation does nothing except to cause pain and joint destruction. **Acetaminophen** may reduce the pain of arthritis, tendinitis, or bursitis, but it won't reduce stiffness the way all other OTC internal analgesics do.

NSAIDs

Ibuprofen, ketoprofen, and **naproxen** are all NSAIDs and can be discussed together, since their actions and side effects are so similar. They are very popular because, although they possess no great advantage over **aspirin** or **acetaminophen** in terms of pain killing and fever reduction, they are much less likely to cause upset stomach than equivalent doses of **aspirin** and they possess the anti-inflammatory effect that **acetaminophen** lacks. Doctors like NSAIDs because high doses—much higher than the OTC maximum—are better tolerated than high doses of aspirin. Higher doses provide greater pain relief. Furthermore, it is at the high end of the dose scale that the anti-inflammatory properties really kick in.

The fact that NSAIDs produce fewer symptoms does not

mean that they are free of side effects. In fact, in some ways the lack of symptoms is a problem, because these products can and do cause *painless* intestinal bleeding and ulcers, including perforated ulcers. NSAIDs are the second highest cause of stomach ulcers, ranking behind infection with the *H. pylori* bacterium.

NSAID manufacturers make claims and counterclaims about the doses and longevity of their products, but there is little objective evidence that one product is better than another, unless your digestive system is rebelling. By trial and error you might find one that is kinder and gentler.

Combination products

Internal analgesics are often combined with other ingredients. Anacin, for instance, combines **aspirin** and **caffeine,** as do a number of other products, although the value of **caffeine** to enhance pain relief is very controversial. Excedrin and Goody's Extra Strength Pain Relief tablets contain **aspirin, acetaminophen,** and **caffeine.** Vanquish includes the same analgesic ingredients plus antacid buffering in the form of **aluminum hydroxide** and **magnesium hydroxide.** BC powders contain **aspirin, salicylamide,** and **caffeine.** There are no products that contain combinations of NSAIDs with any other pain reliever.

Recommendations (internal analgesics)

For general, temporary, and pure pain relief of conditions like headache, use generic **acetaminophen.** It is as effective as any and it is the safest, for both children and adults. If you are not satisfied, try an NSAID.

For menstrual cramps, one of the NSAIDs will prove most helpful. They are so similar you might as well choose a generic form of **ibuprofen.**

If you have ulcers or a history of ulcers and do not want to take **acetaminophen,** you should see your doctor before using anything else. One possibility is to take the prescription drug misoprostol (Cytotec) along with one of the other internal analgesics. It is the only medication that effectively counteracts the damaging effects of NSAIDs on the intestinal tract.

117

If you have kidney disease, consult your doctor before taking any of the NSAIDs.

Don't mix internal analgesics. Take one at a time.

Table 8. OTC internal analgesics

Drug	Inflammation	Pain & fever	Blood thinning	Comments
acetaminophen	–	++	–	C, D
aspirin	++	++	+++	A
ibuprofen	++	++	+	B
ketoprofen	++	++	+	B
magnesium salicylate	++	++	–	B, F
naproxen	++	++	+	B
choline salicylate	++	++	++	E
sodium salicylate	++	++	++	E

–	No effect
+	Fair
++	Good
+++	Better

A	Considerable upset stomach
B	Moderate upset stomach
C	Not useful for menstrual cramps
D	Safe for children
E	Limited availability
F	Take care in kidney disease

External analgesics

If the ideal pain reliever existed it would be something topical, a lotion or cream that you could rub on. It would immediately and completely relieve your discomfort; it would be free of side effects; it would not enter your bloodstream to affect parts of the body where it was not needed; and it would be odorless, greaseless, and inexpensive. The available OTC products, unfortunately, only fulfill one or two of the above requirements, and they do not fulfill them very well. Still, pain is a universal affliction, and internal analgesics are not for everyone. Under certain conditions, giving an external preparation a try might be worthwhile.

External analgesics are usually used to relieve minor muscle and joint pain, such as that due to arthritis, sprains, strains, tendinitis, or bursitis. The FDA-approved wording on the labels of external analgesies also mentions "simple backache." These products do not relieve inflammation at all, but they block the pain.

Most of these products rely on the principle of counterirritation, where one sensation is designed to replace, displace, or counteract another sensation. For example, since the nerves within your knee and the nerves on the skin of your knee share a common pathway, a mild irritation on the skin might override some of the pain impulses from the joint itself. The idea, in effect, is to take your mind off the real pain. Unfortunately, the phenomenon doesn't last very long or work very well.

Counterirritants do feel good when you put them on. There is an initial feeling of coolness, followed by a feeling of heat and sometimes tingling. Your skin might get red. They also smell good, in a medicinal sense. There is no doubt that they are doing something, but the effectiveness of that something is open to question.

For one thing, it is absolutely impossible to devise a good scientific study to see how well counterirritant external analgesics work: test subjects know at once whether they are applying the real stuff or a dummy medication. The placebo effect is bound to be very strong.

For another thing, you don't really need to apply a drug at all to produce counterirritation. Local heat and massage will do the same thing, and part of the treatment with an external analgesic is that you have to rub (massage) it in. The massage, in fact, is often a prominent part of the treatment because it, too, feels good.

The groups and effects of counterirritants are summarized in Table 9.

Table 9. External analgesics

Ingredient	Redness (heat)	Coolness	Irritation
Group A ammonia water methyl salicylate mustard oil phenol turpentine	X		X
Group B camphor menthol		X	
Group C methyl nicotinate	X		
Group D capsaicin			X

Commercial products are available in lots of different combinations and strengths, but some patterns are popular and repeat themselves, for example:

- Absorbine jr. and Pain Patch: **menthol.**
- ArthriCare Triple Medicated Pain Relieving Rub: **methyl salicylate, menthol,** and **methyl nicotinate.**
- Campho-phenique: **camphor** and **phenol.**
- Heet: **methyl salicylate, camphor,** and **capsaicin.**
- Mentholatum Deep Heating Rub, Icy Hot, and BenGay Original: **methyl salicylate** and **menthol.**
- Noxzema Original: **camphor, menthol,** and **phenol.**
- Sloan's Liniment: **turpentine oil** and **capsaicin.**

Although the possible combinations are endless, particularly when different strengths of **menthol, camphor, phenol,** and **methyl salicylate** are used, including more than one ingredient from the same group is probably redundant. There are currently no preparations that contain one ingredient from each of the four categories, but several contain one from each of three.

Capsaicin (Zostrix, Capzasin-P, and others) deserves special mention. It is the newest external analgesic and was initially available only by prescription for the pain that often occurs after an attack of shingles (herpes zoster), a particularly severe type of neuralgia for which no good treatment is available. Since then, it has been used for a variety of conditions, with various results. It is an interesting substance that is the same active ingredient that makes peppers taste hot.

Unlike other counterirritants, **capsaicin** appears to work by removing a chemical called substance P from nerves, thereby making them less able to conduct pain impulses. It is also unlike the others because the best results are seen after several weeks of repeated continual treatment (at least two weeks of applying it three or four times a day). During that time the burning sensation that accompanies treatment will also dissipate. The success rate is around fifty percent, and the treatment can be expensive. **Capsaicin** is available in two strengths, the regular .025 percent and a stronger .075 percent, with the stronger being the more economical.

Trolamine salicylate, unlike the other external analgesics, is not a counterirritant, but acts by increasing levels of salicylate—the active compound in **aspirin**—in tissues. It is found in Aspercreme, Mobisyl, Myoflex, and Sportscreme, and although it has been around for some time, it was only recently approved for use. Unlike the other external analgesics it does not have an aroma nor is there any sensation when it is applied.

Because **trolamine salicylate** is a salicylate (as is **methyl salicylate**), some of the same warnings apply to it as to **aspirin,** and applying large amounts of it can increase salicylate blood levels. Both substances, therefore, should be avoided in those sensitive to salicylates, in pregnancy, and in nursing mothers. They should also not be applied to children or teenagers with symptoms of the flu or chickenpox because of the possibility of inducing Reye's syndrome.

Recommendations (external analgesics)

Although both internal and external analgesics are labelled safe and effective for pain relief, in terms of *relative* safety and efficacy the two types are not comparable. The externals are far safer but also far less effective than their internal counterparts. If you cannot or do not want to use internal analgesics, try the external type.

Of the available remedies, a plain **capsaicin** .075 percent cream is your best bet. Although more expensive than all the others, it isn't messy, doesn't stain, and doesn't smell. Disadvantages include the necessity for frequent applications and the fact that it sometimes doesn't achieve its full effect for as long as six weeks.

If **capsaicin** doesn't seem to help, try **trolamine salicylate** in generic form.

If that doesn't work, try one of the counterirritant combinations, such as Arthricare Triple Medicated Pain Relieving Rub, which contains ingredients from three categories.

If severe burning or irritation develops with any of these, particularly with redness or blisters, stop immediately.

Be particularly careful not to touch your eyes, nose, or genital skin after application.

Of the counterirritants, avoid those with high concentrations of **camphor** and **turpentine.**

Never use any external analgesic in conjunction with a heating pad or hot water bottle.

23

POISONING

Poisonings and overdoses are a significant cause of illness, coma, and death, especially in children. They are also a frequent cause of calls to hospitals, emergency rooms, pharmacies, doctors' offices, and poison control centers.

In poisoning, time is of the essence. You have no greater ally than a poison control center. Of course, if the person is unconscious or semi-conscious there is nothing you can do at home. In this case, call 911 immediately or take the person to an emergency room immediately.

When calling the poison control center, the more information you can provide the better. This includes not only the name and amount of what the victim took, but his or her weight, general health, and other drugs or medications that may have been taken at the same time. It is also important to note any symptoms, such as the general level of consciousness and any abnormal behavior.

The person you speak to may reassure you that nothing needs to be done or the person may give you instructions for emergency treatment. For example, if a caustic like lye has been ingested, you may be told to give the patient some milk to drink to immediately counteract the damage.

In some cases, you may be instructed to get the patient to vomit by using **ipecac,** the only OTC drug approved for this purpose. In order to use it quickly, of course, it is best to have it on hand to begin with, which requires some planning.

Ipecac can generally be given to *alert* adults and to children over the age of six months, unless they have ingested a strong caustic, certain oil-containing substances, or sharp objects such as glass. **Ipecac** works best with a lot of fluid. Any fluids are fine, but clear liquids are best because they do not interfere with the examination of the vomit for pills or capsules. **Ipecac** also works best if a person is active; patients should be encouraged to move about. If vomiting does not take place within thirty minutes, another dose of **ipecac** can be given. At no time during this process should the patient be left alone.

If you have been instructed both to take **ipecac** *and* go to an emergency room, bring along a bucket or other container for the patient to vomit into. Don't wait for vomiting to occur before setting out for the hospital.

Some hospitals and poison centers prefer the use of **activated charcoal** to **ipecac**. **Activated charcoal** does not induce vomiting but, rather, adsorbs toxic substances so that they do not enter the bloodstream. **Activated charcoal** can adsorb up to ten times the number of chemical molecules as there are charcoal molecules. In some instances, both **ipecac** and **activated charcoal** are used, the charcoal being administered only after vomiting has taken place. **Activated charcoal** is very safe. Large and repeated doses can be taken without ill effects. It has been shown to be effective in reducing the ill effects of many drugs and toxic substances.

Although there is no reason why you cannot take or administer **activated charcoal** at home, it is usually not practical because most children can't be made to take an adequate dose. It has to be mixed with water to form a sludge and it doesn't taste good. As a result, it is usually given in a hospital, sometimes through a tube inserted into the stomach. There are also times when a mixture of **activated charcoal** and a laxative is given, but again this is almost always a hospital procedure.

It should be noted that **activated charcoal** is not at all the same as burnt toast, nor is it the ingredient in the so-called universal antidote, which consists of burnt toast, strong tea, and **magnesium hydroxide** (milk of magnesia). The universal antidote, by the way, is worthless and should *never* be used in poisoning.

Recommendations

Prevention is better than treatment. Keep medicine, drugs, vitamins, and household chemicals out of reach of children. This includes medications you may keep in your handbag.

Throw out all medicines that are outdated or no longer needed.

Paste the telephone number of your nearest poison control center (see Appendix IV) on all phones and make sure your babysitter knows how to call this number.

Keep ipecac on hand.

24

SKIN, HAIR, AND NAILS

Although skin, hair, and nail remedies comprise a substantial part of the OTC market, it is not always easy to know what you should use in a given situation. This is because skin rashes, despite how easy they are to see and examine, can be very mysterious and confusing, even to specialists. Being constipated, having diarrhea, or suffering from a headache will automatically lead you to the correct area of the drugstore, but having something wrong with your skin can be a daunting problem, given the hundreds of possible skin diseases. And in addition to contending with the bombardment of advice you get from advertisers, you also often have to evaluate the opinions of your beautician, cosmetologist, and mother.

Something as simple as dry skin can pose problems. Dry skin of the feet, for example, can actually be a type of athlete's foot. Dry skin of the elbows can be a type of psoriasis. Dry skin of the scalp, eyebrows, and sides of the nose can be the condition known as seborrhea. Dry patches on the forehead can be a precancerous skin condition known as solar keratoses. So in order to get the proper medication, you have to make the proper diagnosis, and this is best done by a doctor.

There are times, however, when it might be appropriate to select a skin remedy on your own, either because you've had the condition before or you are fairly certain about what's going on.

Acne

Although acne is the easiest skin disease to diagnose yourself, the individual lesions themselves can look very different from one another. There may be whiteheads (small white bumps), blackheads (black spots within the pore), pustules (red pimples with a white dot of pus), cysts (fluid filled sacs), papules (small red bumps without a drop of pus), or nodules (large red bumps). Doctors classify acne by the main types of lesion and also by general severity into mild, moderate, or severe (cystic) cases. If you consider that even one pimple can be considered to be acne, then it is probably a universal affliction.

Acne is an inflammation in hair follicles, which are sometimes called pores, the tiny holes in your skin through which hair grows. Although the precise nature of the condition is not known, it is likely that germs (a bacterium known as *P. acnes*) present in the follicle are the main problem. In order to grow, the germs need skin oils—which accumulate considerably around puberty—and they actually change the composition of the oils. The germs, the changed oils, and the response of the body to the infection then inflame the follicle, causing an acne blemish. This process, although mostly present in adolescence, may occur at any time.

A number of things to keep in mind:

- There is no scientific evidence that foods have anything to do with acne.
- There is no evidence that dehydration is to blame. Drinking lots of water or other fluids will only make you urinate more.
- There is no evidence that acne comes from not washing your face enough.

These myths persist, and although they may appear harmless, the problem with approaching your problem by trying to adjust your life is that it will only lead to frustration and a guilt trip. Acne is from bad luck, not bad habits.

Emotional stress can trigger a flare of acne. Breaking up with your boyfriend or girlfriend, taking final exams, preparing for your wedding, or getting fired from your job can definitely make it worse.

One way to approach acne is to forget all about it and let it run its course. It is true that most people outgrow it, although one can't predict when. But besides the social and psychological problems it causes (and these can be considerable), there is the danger of scarring, which can be extremely hard if not impossible to treat.

The following four ingredients, all topical (external), are available OTC for acne: **benzoyl peroxide, salicylic acid, sulfur,** and **resorcinol.** Unfortunately, unless you have acne that is mild or moderate in severity, you're not likely to be helped much by them.

Benzoyl peroxide, which is widely available in various strengths and forms, is the most effective of these. It is also the one dermatologists use most often, although usually in conjunction with other medications. It is, however, currently being investigated by the FDA because of the possibility that it may promote (not *cause*) skin cancer from sunlight. The fact is, however, that anything that irritates the skin—and **benzoyl peroxide** can cause severe skin irritation—may make one more susceptible to skin cancer, because the natural defenses are decreased.

Salicylic acid is available in pads, solutions, and cleansers. It is a keratolytic, something that disrupts the top layer of skin (the keratin) and mostly assists other medications to work by helping them to penetrate through this firm layer. The **salicylic acid** present in acne medications is weaker than the **salicylic acid** present in wart removers.

Sulfur and **resorcinol** should be thought of together since this is the way they seem to work the best. **Resorcinol,** in fact, is only approved for acne when it is mixed with **sulfur.** Both have effects against bacteria and are keratolytic.

Since acne fluctuates greatly in intensity it is impossible to decide for yourself over a short period of time whether a medication is effective or not. In other words, if you start applying an OTC medication today and your acne is remarkably better tomorrow, it definitely wasn't the medicine that did it, unless your face got so red that your pimples blended in with your background skin color.

One strategy for self-treatment of acne is to try all of the available OTC medications for a period of time. If improvement is satisfactory, stick with it. If not, you should seek medical attention.

The difficulty with this approach is that if you try to apply all the medications at once your skin will get quite irritated, developing redness, scaling, stinging, burning, or itching. Some individuals are very sensitive to these ingredients and cannot use them at all. For this reason, it is best to stay with one preparation in its lowest strength for a week or two. If you can tolerate it, add another until you are using all of them.

When you have gotten to the point of using all available OTC products you will be putting something on three times a day: once for **benzoyl peroxide**, once for **salicylic acid**, and once for **sulfur** and **resorcinol**. In the morning, for example, you might apply a 2.5 percent **benzoyl peroxide** such as Clear by Design or On the Spot (although you should not apply acne medicines only on the spot, since once a blemish appears, it is too late for externally applied medications to help). In the afternoon, you could use a .5 percent **salicylic acid** pad, gel, or liquid such as Clean & Clear Invisible Blemish Treatment for Sensitive Skin or Oxy Deep Cleansing for Sensitive Skin. Before bed, a 5 percent **sulfur** and 2 percent **resorcinol** combination product such as Rezamid or Sulforcin should be applied. Pay attention to the percentages so as not to get overly irritated. Do this regularly, treating the entire area that is breaking out. Stop everything if your face gets even slightly irritated and wait a day or two for it to calm down. During this time wash the areas you are treating with a mild soap such as Dove two times a day. Use lukewarm water and your hands rather than a washcloth or abrasive device. Don't scrub too hard.

If you can tolerate this regimen, you can increase the strengths of the various medications, going to a 5 percent **benzoyl peroxide**, for example, and to a 2 percent **salicylic acid**. If this program doesn't work in about three months, it is not likely to work. You should judge your response in terms of large blocks of time. The occasional flare-ups don't mean much, and the only way to know if you are being helped is to look at the big picture.

Studies show that there is no great advantage of one external acne medication over another; they all seem to be about equal. This applies to prescription as well as nonprescription drugs. What they can't compete with, however, are prescription *oral* antibiotics, and for this you need a doctor. The most severe cases can be controlled with the prescription vitamin A derivative called Accutane.

Keep in mind the following points:

- All OTC acne products are designed to prevent new lesions from occurring, not to treat the ones that have already appeared.
- Don't apply moisturizers where you have acne. Any place else on your skin is fine.
- Don't pick. Pimples can be squeezed to get the pus out only if there is a white point on the surface. If it is not there, do not manipulate the pimple.

Athlete's foot

Athlete's foot refers to an infection with ringworm fungus, a type of germ that is very different from bacteria and viruses. It is so common that in practice, unfortunately, any rash on the foot is likely to be called athlete's foot, and it is quite easy to treat oneself for the wrong condition over a long time.

Rashes of the feet generally fall into one of three categories, athlete's foot, eczema, and contact dermatitis. Although they can all look alike—and even dermatologists have problems differing them sometimes—they can usually be distinguished.

The easiest foot rash to rule out is contact dermatitis, which is an allergy to some ingredient used in shoe manufacturing, such as leather tanning agents, glues, or rubber. The eruption will almost always show up worst on the tops of your feet, particularly on the big toe, and will not involve the spaces between the toes. If you don't wear the footgear that you are allergic to, the rash goes away. When you wear the shoes again, the rash comes back. The best treatment is to get rid of the shoes, although if you keep the shoes *very* dry you will decrease the problem.

Eczema (also called atopic dermatitis or dyshidrosis) of the feet can be more difficult to diagnose. It is usually, but not always, associated with eczema elsewhere and is often found in families with a history of multiple allergies, hives, asthma, or hay fever. If athlete's foot remedies have usually been unsuccessful in your case, especially if the rash tends to come and go mysteriously, you may very well have eczema. Furthermore, foot eczema is often associated with hand eczema; if you have a chronic rash on both hands and both feet you almost certainly have a type of eczema. Children with foot rashes, by the way, usually have eczema, not athelete's foot. Treatment, if the case is mild, is with **hydrocortisone** creams or ointments, but if the case is severe you will need a prescription medication.

Athlete's foot itself can look different in different people. Sometimes it is red and scaling over the entire surface of the foot, like a mocassin, and is mistaken for dry skin. Sometimes it consists of small firm blisters. Sometimes the spaces between the toes—particularly between the fourth and little toes—are cracked or whitish.

When the toenails are infected with a fungus they become thick, yellow, and crumbly. The nails then act as a reservoir for the fungus, and no external antifungal product, either OTC or prescription, will reverse it. To clear the fungus from the nail you need an oral prescription medication.

Although often considered trivial, athlete's foot can be troublesome in diabetics and those with poor circulation. The cracks in the skin may help introduce bacteria that can cause serious infections.

There are four OTC ingredients available to treat athlete's foot fungus: **undecylenate, tolnaftate, clotrimazole,** and **miconazole.** Most are available in a variety of creams, ointments, sprays, powders, soaps, and foams.

Undecylenate (also known as undecylenic acid, zinc undecylenate, or 10-undecenoic acid), is present in the Desenex and Cruex product lines. It is of moderate cost but not very effective. Also, some people find the odor objectionable. In general, there is little to recommend it.

Tolnaftate, available in Aftate, Tinactin, Ting, and generics, is moderately expensive and somewhat more effective than **undecylenate.** Unfortunately, it is not an antibacterial, and it is sometimes ineffective when bacteria are growing in addition to the fungus, as often happens between the toes. For prevention of athlete's foot in those susceptible to it, the powder form is a convenient way to keep the fungal organisms under control.

Clotrimazole (Lotrimin, Mycelex) and miconazole (Lotrimin AF, Micatin) are the best OTC antifungals on the market. They are both in the azole class of fungus-fighters, and are practically interchangeable. Lotrimin AF cream, for instance, contains clotrimazole, whereas Lotrimin AF powder has miconazole. Although more expensive, clotrimazole and miconazole are also definitely more effective than the other antifungal ingredients and have a broader spectrum of activity, killing yeasts as well as true fungi. It is not always easy to tell a yeast infection from a true fungus infection of the skin, so this shotgun approach to treatment is sometimes more effective. Other advantages to the azoles is that they have antibacterial qualities and tend not to irritate the skin. If you can afford them, they are well worth the extra cost.

Susceptibility to most diseases, even infectious ones, can be partly hereditary, and some people are more sensitive to athlete's foot than others. Thus, even after cure, it is common for athlete's foot to recur. If you are particularly susceptible, opportunities to catch the germ are innumberable: at the gym, in motel and hotel rooms, at the pool, even in your own home. To the certainty of death, taxes, and bifocals, therefore, we should add fungus in the shower stall.

Suggestions:

- If you have athlete's foot but your nails are clear you should be able to cure it by using either miconazole or clotrimazole twice a day, faithfully, for six weeks straight. If it isn't gone by that time the rash isn't a fungus or a yeast.
- After it is cured, use a powder containing tolnaftate, such as Zeasorb-AF prophylactically and indefinitely to prevent recurrence. At the first sign of recurrence, treat yourself again.
- If your nails are involved but you don't want to take an oral prescription medicine use the miconazole or clotrimazole on and around your nails indefinitely (for the rest of your life) to prevent a recurrence.
- Don't wear the same shoes more than two days in a row, especially if your feet sweat a lot. Wooden,

132

not metal, shoe trees help by absorbing moisture from the inside of your shoes and keeping them dry.

Table 10. OTC antifungal athlete's foot medications

Product	Cost	Effectiveness
Undecylenate	$$	+
Tolnaftate	$$	++
Miconazole	$$$	+++
Clotrimazole	$$$	+++

Dandruff, seborrhea, and psoriasis

Dandruff, seborrhea, and psoriasis are often lumped together because they all tend to cause excessive flaking of the scalp and because OTC shampoos are labelled as being good for all of them. Another similarity is that nobody really knows what causes these conditions, except for genetic tendencies. But there are differences, which are detailed in Table 11. The table also describes features of eczema (atopic dermatitis), which can also cause scalp itching and flaking.

Table 11. Dandruff, seborrhea, psoriasis, and eczema symptoms

	Dandruff	Seborrhea	Psoriasis	Eczema
other locations besides scalp	none	eyebrows, behind ears, along the sides of the nose, central chest, armpits, groin	elbows, knees, navel, upper crease of skin between buttocks; may be scattered over entire body	crease of elbows, backs of knees, around eyes, hands, and feet; may be scattered over entire body
redness	no	yes	yes	yes
itching	+/−	+/++	scalp ++; other locations +/−	++++

In practice, any OTC dandruff shampoo can be used to treat any of these conditions. In general, however, simple dandruff is the most amenable to treatment, followed by seborrhea and psoriasis. Psoriasis can be so stubborn, in fact, that it resists even potent prescription medications.

Available shampoos contain one of the following five

active ingredients: **pyrithione zinc, selenium sulfide, salicylic acid, sulfur,** or **coal tar.** The **salicylic acid** and **sulfur** are often combined together.

Pyrithione zinc in 1 percent strength is contained in most Head & Shoulders products, but there are stronger ones with 2 percent of it, such as DHS Zinc and Sebulon.

Selsun Blue is the best known **selenium sulfide** shampoo, although Head & Shoulders Intensive Treatment also has it. These are both 1 percent concentrations. A 2.5 percent strength is available by prescription and is more effective.

Denorex and Tegrin both contain **coal tar,** but there are many other shampoos that contain it as well. Although there are various strengths, the real differences between the products have to do more with cosmetic acceptability, because **coal tar** in its crude state is messy and smelly.

Salicylic acid and **sulfur** are best used in combination products such as Meted and Sebulex, but some shampoos contain only the **salicylic acid.**

Finding a shampoo that will keep your dandruff under control is a matter of trial and error. The best advice is to stick with one product and use it every other day, keeping it in contact with your scalp for about three minutes. If it doesn't work within six weeks of use it probably won't, and you should go on to something else. Try **pyrithione zinc** first, followed by **selenium sulfide,** then **coal tar,** and lastly a **sulfur** and **salicylic acid** combination. Once you get your dandruff under control, decrease the frequency of shampooing, alternating with a non-medicated shampoo.

Most of the time the symptoms of dandruff are clear. There are two things to be aware of, however:

- Ringworm (a fungus infection) of the scalp can look like simple dandruff, especially in children.
- Very stubborn dandruff, or dandruff in which red patches extend onto your forehead, may be seborrhea or psoriasis.

Seborrhea (or seborrheic dermatitis) is a very common condition that is often mistaken for dry skin. It can affect not only the scalp, but also the ears (particularly behind the ears), eyebrows, sides of the nose, cheeks, middle of the chest, armpits, and groin. Unlike simple dandruff, seborrhea is red and can be very itchy. When it occurs in its most common pattern, along the eyebrows and sides of the nose, it is often mistaken for dryness in the so-called T-zone.

Besides trying an OTC shampoo for dandruff, you might use **hydrocortisone** in the cream form to bring down inflammation. (The ointment form is too messy to be used in hairy areas.) To apply the cream to the scalp, dab a bit on your finger, part your hair, and run your finger along the exposed skin.

Many people who have had seborrhea for years suddenly may show up with symptoms of psoriasis. Indeed, there is some evidence that they may be two forms of the same underlying problem, one mild and one more severe.

Most of the time, you will need a doctor to diagnose psoriasis, although it is usually fairly characteristic: thick red patches with a silvery scale most often on the elbows, knees, scalp, and body. It is a very common disease, affecting perhaps two to three percent of the population.

Since the tendency to psoriasis is hereditary, there is no cure, and the best one can hope for is to be able to control it. The object of treatment is to allow you to at least live with the symptoms without too much discomfort or embarrassment. Understand that this may not be and often is not total clearing. In general, the more you can stand, psychologically, the better off you will be. There is nothing to be gained by aggressive treatment unless you are signficantly troubled by your condition. Don't expect miracles with OTC drugs; some cases are so severe that even prescription medications have a hard time. One good rule is never to buy a psoriasis nostrum hawked on TV or the radio.

For mild psoriasis on skin other than the scalp you should first see if you can get by with a simple moisturizer, such as plain **petrolatum** (petroleum jelly). This might be sufficient to keep the scales down. If this doesn't do the trick, try **hydrocortisone** in the ointment (greasy) form two times a day. You'll generally have to use this for about a month to see if it works.

Coal tar is an ancient remedy that sometimes helps psoriasis. As its name implies, in natural form it is black, gooey, and smells bad, so that drug manufacturers have spent considerable time and money trying to find cosmetically acceptable forms of it. At present, the best tolerated ones are gel forms, such as Estar, although gels can dry the skin. If drying is a problem, an ointment (grease) such as MG217 for Psoriasis may be more appealing. Another way to avoid drying is to use the ingredient as a bath or body oil, such as Balnetar or Neutrogena T/Derm, although if these are added to the water itself they will make the tub slippery.

Salicylic acid by itself or in combination with **sulfur** and **coal tar** is also present in some products. It helps by reducing scale and making the skin more permeable to other medications. Scalpicin and P&S contain a liquid form of **salicylic acid** that is more convenient to apply to the scalp.

Psoriasis usually gets worse in the winter and improves in the summer, particularly in the sun. If you find ultraviolet light helpful, using one of the **coal tar** products will enhance the effect. Make certain, however, to cover non-involved areas with clothing or sunscreens and be careful never to get burned.

Although psoriasis usually doesn't itch very much, on the scalp it can be very annoying. Since it doesn't do well if irritated, make certain you don't get into a scratching and picking habit.

The Psoriasis Foundation is a non-profit organization which helps patients and doctors deal with the disease. People who suffer from psoriasis are often the butt of jokes, but psoriasis in its severe forms can be disabling. It is possible to have virtually one hundred percent of your skin red, flaking, and peeling.

Deodorants and antiperspirants

If you usually use an antiperspirant and make the mistake of buying a simple deodorant some day, you will know about it soon enough. Deodorants do nothing for perspiration and very little for underarm body odor.

Most antiperspirants contain an aluminum-zirconium compound or **aluminum chlorohydrate** as the active ingredient. If this is not sufficient and you are still perspiring, you can obtain **aluminum chloride** as an OTC liquid in the form of Certain Dri. It tends to sting and may produce skin irritation, but in general it is more effective than commercial antiperspirants. It can be used also for excessive sweating of the hands and feet. A stronger, 20 percent **aluminum chloride** (Drysol) is available by prescription for really copious perspiration.

Diaper rash

Diaper rash is caused by moisture, rubbing, urine, feces, heat, and sweating. It can occur not only in infants but in the elderly who are incontinent.

Diapers are highly unnatural contrivances to begin with; we were meant to eliminate our waste and leave it in the woods, not to enclose it in plastic and wrap it around our bottoms. The most important thing to remember about true diaper rash is that it is caused by prolonged contact with wet diapers. If the skin is kept perfectly dry and open to the air, the problem disappears on its own. No amount of cream or powder can take the place of a soft, clean diaper.

Although there is some controversy, disposable diapers are probably better than cloth, and the vast majority of mothers—around eight out of ten—agree, buying Huggies or Pampers. The best kind are the ones labelled "super absorbable." If you do use cloth, you should either employ a commercial diaper service (if you can find one) or soak and disinfect the diapers prior to washing them yourself; doing them in the regular laundry isn't enough.

Besides changing diapers frequently, you should avoid plastic pants, which only tend to aggravate the problem. When you cleanse the diaper area use a very small amount of a mild soap, such as Dove, and rinse well with lukewarm water. Dry with a soft towel or a hair dryer set on low.

There are many OTC powders, ointments, pastes, gels, and lotions sold for preventing and treating diaper rash. In general, these consist of a protectant and an antiseptic.

Protectants reduce friction and coat the skin to prevent irritation. OTC protectants include such things as **petrolatum** (petroleum jelly), **zinc oxide, cod-liver oil, mineral oil, oatmeal, lanolin, cocoa butter,** and **silicone.** Powders have protectant qualities but also absorb moisture. They usually contain **cornstarch, talc, magnesium stearate, calcium carbonate,** or **kaolin.**

Antiseptics, which kill germs, include **benzalkonium chloride, benzethonium chloride, undecylenate, chloroxylenol, methylbenzethonium chloride,** and **cetylpyridinium chloride.**

Although millions of babies have had such products patted and rubbed onto their buttocks, there is little to recommend one product over another or one ingredient over another, and they may actually do more harm than good. One difficulty is that they can cake up and be very hard to remove. At the very least they should never take the place of scrupulous cleanliness. They should also only be used to prevent diaper rash, not treat it. Don't put these products on raw, open, or oozing skin.

If your baby is prone to diaper rash and you can't seem to stop it, try dusting with a little **cornstarch,** being careful not to let the baby breathe in any particles. Contrary to some opinions, **cornstarch** doesn't support the growth of germs and is safer than **talc.** It also absorbs much more moisture than **talc.**

You might also use plain **zinc oxide** paste, which contains **petrolatum** and **cornstarch** in addition to **zinc oxide,** or plain **petrolatum.** To remove them adequately from the skin you will need something like **mineral oil** or cold cream.

There are other skin conditions that can affect the diaper area, such as eczema, yeast infections, bacterial infections (impetigo), and seborrhea; if the rash is stubborn, see a doctor.

Dry skin

As was mentioned above, it is fairly common to think you have dry skin when it is actually something else entirely. Nonetheless, little harm can come from applying a commercial moisturizer to such problems; the worst that can happen is that the correct treatment might be delayed. As a rule, if the dry skin—or what you think is dry skin—doesn't go away nicely with a moisturizer within a couple of weeks, you should see a doctor.

True dry skin almost always shows up first—and worst—on the lower legs, arms, and trunk of the body. Sometimes it gets so bad that the skin actually develops cracks and fissures. In severe cases scales like fish skin (ichthyosis) may be seen. Red, coin-shaped patches can also appear and itch intensely. Dry skin of the face is rare, although some flaking and a feeling of tightness is common after washing or bathing, or after being chapped by cold weather or the wind. Dry skin is considerably worse in the winter, and often is only seen then. The elderly suffer from it more than the young.

For those whose skin dries out in the winter (winter eczema or winter itch) there are two things that will almost always solve the problem: a short shower followed by a moisturizing lotion. Use a kitchen timer to learn to take a three minute shower—it's faster than you think—with water as cool or lukewarm as you can stand it. Use a mild soap like Dove. Towel off and rub the dry areas with a moisturizer while they are still a little damp.

The term moisturizer deserves some discussion. Although the name is thrown around loosely in consumer literature, it is not actually recognized by pharmacologists, dermatologists, or the FDA. What are usually referred to as moisturizers are technically emollients. An emollient softens the skin and forms a greasy or oily barrier to prevent water loss. Thus, it doesn't actually moisturize, that is, add water to the skin, but only helps to hold on to what is already there. The real name for something that adds moisture is humectant.

To add to the confusion, there are also demulcents, which soothe, and protectants, which protect. A number of ingredients fall into more than one category, and distinctions, as is often the case, are often blurred.

To make some sense out of the host of ingredients you will see on most commercial moisturizers, however, it is necessary to impose some order on the situation. For instance, Keri Silky Smooth Formula lists the following: water, **petrolatum, glycerin,** dimethicone, steareth-2, cetyl alcohol, **benzyl alcohol,** laureth-23, magnesium aluminum silicate, carbomer, fragrance, sodium hydroxide, and quaternium-15.

Eucerin Plus Creme contains water, **mineral oil, urea, magnesium stearate,** ceresin, polyglyceryl-3, diiosostearate, sodium lactate, isopropyl palmitate, **benzyl alcohol,** panthenol, bisabolol, **lanolin, alcohol,** and **magnesium sulfate.**

Unless you're a cosmetic chemist you shouldn't make any attempt to understand what everything is doing in there. In fact, if you're like most people, the only thing you recognized in both lists is the water, which is very interesting because it is also the most important thing. The major ingredients other than water will fall into one of the following categories:

- emollients and protectants
- humectants
- keratolytics
- alpha-hydroxy acids

Emollients and protectants

Most ingredients in this category feel greasy or oily. The general principle in most commercial moisturizers is to whip water and an emollient together; the water goes into the skin and the emollient keeps it there. Most commonly you will find **petrolatum** (petroleum jelly), **lanolin, mineral oil, allantoin,** or **silicone** (dimethicone) listed. Of these, **petrolatum** is the most effective and **silicone** the least effective. In fact, if you were to soak your skin with water to saturate it (which takes a few minutes) and then apply plain petroleum jelly, you would be moisturizing your skin in the most effective way possible. Most people won't do this, however, because it is a nuisance and because it is messy. The manufacture of moisturizers, in fact, is a balancing act between what works well and what feels good. As a rule, though, the products that feel the most elegant are also the least effective.

Humectants

These true moisturizers are usually represented by **glycerin,** although **propylene glycol,** and **sorbitol** are sometimes used. They work by drawing in and absorbing water. In the low concentrations present in most moisturizers they work well, but in higher concentrations they may irritate and actually dehydrate the skin.

Keratolytics

The major ingredient in this category is **urea.** Keratolytics decompose keratin, the protein that forms the bulk of the topmost or horny layer of the skin as well as the bulk of hair and nails. In very high concentrations, in fact, **urea** can be used in a paste to remove toenails. When placed on a diseased nail and taped in place it soons turns the nail into a soft and crumbly mass.

Keratin is the substance that allows the skin to function as a barrier and is analgous to the bark of a tree. In low strengths **urea** can decompose this layer just enough to allow water to penetrate easily, and it is very effective for this purpose. Unfortunately, it also has a tendency to sting if applied to open or raw spots.

Alpha-hydroxy acids

These are the newest moisturizer ingredients and have become very popular both because of intense marketing and because they have the cachet of being natural. How they work is not known, but they may be partly humectant, partly keratolytic, and partly something else. These substances include **lactic acid**, **citric acid**, **malic acid**, and **glycolic acid**. The only prescription moisturizer, Lac-Hydrin 12 percent, contains **lactic acid** (in addition to water, **glycerin, mineral oil,** and **propylene glycol**) but weaker strengths are freely available. High concentrations can produce significant irritation and can be used as chemical peels under medical supervision. Alpha-hydroxy acids are discussed more fully in the section on wrinkles in this chapter.

Recommendations

Although most ingredients won't give you trouble, there are people who get very irritated by things like **lanolin, propylene glycol, alpha-hydroxy acids,** and certain preservatives. **Mineral oil** and **petrolatum** can cause a type of acne. So if you don't need it, don't apply it. Entirely too much moisturizer is consumed in the United States. Many people use it because they think they are supposed to. Moisturizers do not prevent wrinkling or aging unless they also contain sunscreen, in which case the effect is entirely due to the sunscreen.

If you do need a moisturizer, buy whatever is on sale and use it right after a quick (three minute) shower. If it works well, stick with it. If it doesn't, look at the label. If it doesn't contain **petrolatum** first or second on its list of ingredients, buy the next less expensive one that does. If that one is unacceptable, try one with **urea** or **lactic acid**. Four or five tries on your own is plenty; after that it's time to see a doctor. A physical exam might be in order and possibly some lab tests to rule out an underactive thyroid or a skin condition other than simple dryness.

There is no evidence that drinking eight glasses of water or liquid a day will keep your skin moist or benefit your skin in any way whatsoever. Your skin can become dry from dehydration, it is true, but this is almost always from prolonged vomiting or diarrhea, a high fever, or heat stroke, not from simply forgetting to drink liquids. If you are this dehydrated, the other symptoms of dehydration will far outweigh your dry skin. Common dry skin is not treatable with anything oral. Using a humidifier or having lots of wide-leafed plants around inside the house will increase the humidity somewhat, but only enough to make a difference to the mucous membranes in your nose and throat, not your skin.

Eczema

Eczema is probably the most difficult skin disease to recognize, since it can look very different in different people and even looks very different in the same person at different stages of life. How it looks also depends on its severity, the color of your skin, and what part of your body is affected.

Eczema is extremely common. For example, you probably have a form of eczema if:

- your skin dries out every winter
- your hands get chapped easily
- you have a problem with redness, scaling, and itching around your eyes that comes and goes
- you have a problem that looks like ringworm but doesn't clear up when you use ringworm medicines
- you get poison ivy every summer even though you don't touch it
- you seem to be allergic to everything

142

- you have athlete's foot that doesn't clear up when you use athlete's foot medications

Strictly speaking, eczema is not an allergy, although many people with eczema also have hay-fever, allergies, or asthma. It is best thought of as an inherited tendency toward sensitive skin. What you inherit is not the disease, but a susceptibility to it. Once you have that predisposition, various events can trigger a flare.

Some people have a distinct pattern to their eczema. Some start to have trouble every October or November when the air dries out. Others predictably worsen in the summer with heat and perspiration. In some, the pattern is one in winter, for instance scaling, thickening, and cracking of the hands, and another in the summer, for instance redness and itching around the eyes and neck. In some, the disease only flares up when the seasons change, in others, only during the pollen seasons in the spring and summer and when their hay fever allergies kick up. Some people with eczema experience their flare-ups only when they are under emotional stress, and because of this, eczema is sometimes called neurodermatitis, although that term has largely fallen into disuse.

More important than the word that's used to describe the condition is what to do about it if you have it. For this, you have to decide whether your eczema is in the acute stage or the chronic stage. Acute *(wet)* eczema blisters, weeps, and oozes fluid. Chronic *(dry)* eczema is red, scaly, or leathery.

For acute eczema, the best thing is a compress. This can be as simple as plain lukewarm tap water on a soft cotton cloth such as an old pillowcase or handkerchief. Soak the cloth, wring it out, and place it on the affected area for fifteen to thirty minutes three or four times a day. Stop when the skin has become sufficiently dry.

A greater drying effect can be obtained with **aluminum acetate** solution, also called Burow's solution. This is available as a powder you can mix yourself in Bluboro or Domeboro. These compresses are also good for helping to dry poison ivy blisters or those from chickenpox or shingles. As an alternative, **witch hazel** can be applied directly to an acute irritation three or four times a day.

Compresses and soaks are not good, however, for chronic,

dry, scaling eczema, or eczema that has been treated with compresses until it has become dry. In fact, they make these conditions worse. Chronic eczema needs lubrication in the form of **petrolatum** (petroleum jelly) or any commercial moisturizer or the anti inflammatory **hydrocortisone.**

The change in availability of **hydrocortisone** from prescription to OTC status, which occurred in 1980, is one of the more significant developments in the ability to treat skin ailments OTC. In 1991 the FDA further liberalized the decision with the approval of stronger one-percent products.

Hydrocortisone is very similar to an essential hormone produced naturally in all humans, called cortisol. It is also a steroid, although not the type that athletes use to build muscles. If given internally in large doses it can have many side effects, but the result of external application is different. What **hydrocortisone** does is reduce inflammation—redness, swelling, scaling, and itching. It is indicated when the skin is inflamed *in the absence of infection,* which is usually the case in chronic eczema.

The labelling on **hydrocortisone** OTC is supposed to include the following words: "For the temporary relief of minor skin irritations, itching, and rashes due to eczema, dermatitis, insect bites, poison ivy, poison oak, poison sumac, soaps, detergents, cosmetics, and jewelry, and for itchy genital and anal areas."

Dermatologists use similar, but much stronger, external steroids as a mainstay in the treatment of numerous skin diseases, but it is possible to use OTC **hydrocortisone** effectively if your condition is mild and you're not in a frenzied itch-scratch cycle.

The most effective **hydrocortisone** preparations are those in ointment (greasy) forms. Although ointments are messier to apply than the cream forms, they definitely work better and are more economical because they spread better. One-percent **hydrocortisone** ointments include: Cortaid Maximum Strength Ointment, Cortizone-10 Ointment, Lanacort 10 ointment, and generics.

The use of such an ointment will work only to a certain point. Eczema will continue or even worsen if one continues to rub or scratch. No matter what the trigger for a flare-up of eczema, the main cause for its persistance is the irritation caused by scratching. The consequence is a cycle in which the act of scratching leads to further irritation and widening of the zone of involvement, so that the eruption appears to spread.

It is next to impossible to consciously will yourself not to scratch if you have a tendency to eczema. If a child or a spouse is suffering it is tempting to tell them not to scratch, but this only leads to frustration all around. Some people use hot water to overcome the sensation. This works temporarily but inevitably makes everything worse. It is far better to "cheat" with the **hydrocortisone** a little and apply it more frequently for relief. It may be helpful to remember that it is physically impossible for any itch to be constant; the nerves always go into a resting phase after a time.

Eczema may also be helped by an antihistamine, particularly if you are having trouble sleeping at night because of itching. You can take one of the less sedating ingredients such as **chlorpheniramine** (Chlor-Trimeton) during the day and a more sedating antihistamine such as **diphenhydramine** (Benadryl) shortly before bedtime.

If these measures don't work, you will need to see a doctor for a stronger prescription topical steroid or even an oral steroid, such as prednisone. A topical antihistamine (doxepin), available by prescription, may also provide relief.

Hair loss

There is only one OTC ingredient you should consider for baldness: **minoxidil** (Rogaine and generics). Everything else is worthless. It is not known how **minoxidil** works, but it is probably by direct stimulation of the hair root in the hair follicle.

Minoxidil is only for common baldness (also called androgenetic baldness), a condition due to a combination of heredity and the effects of male hormones such as testosterone. Common baldness is also known as pattern baldness, because it tends to affect some areas more than others. In men, these areas are the crown of the scalp and the front of the scalp; in women, the entire top of the scalp tends to thin out. In both sexes, the hair on the sides and back of the head usually remains thick and full.

Hair loss that is much more extensive or patchy is probably not common baldness and needs medical evaluation. Thyroid problems, iron deficiency, and many drugs (such as **aspirin, ibuprofen, ketoprofen,** or **naproxen**) may cause significant hair loss. If you have a scalp condition, this should also be investigated, since it may be related to the hair loss (most often, however, it is not).

The big question about minoxidil is, does it work?

The answer is that about half of men, and a somewhat smaller percentage of women, note some regrowth of hair, although it is often just a bit of peach fuzz. Nine out of ten times, however, minoxidil will halt further progression of hair loss, but you'll have to use it for the rest of your life. Thus, most people will continue to look the same while using minoxidil, and you won't be able to tell, five or ten or fifteen years down the road, whether you would have stayed that way naturally or if the minoxidil actually did work. The only way to know for certain would be for your identical twin brother or sister to engage in the experiment at the same time, with only one of you using the drug.

If you stop using minoxidil after a period of time you will revert to the way you would have looked normally. This will take a year or two, and although it might be alarming to lose that much hair that quickly, you won't be any worse off.

When minoxidil was switched from prescription to OTC status the price went down dramatically. What used to cost about sixty dollars a month now costs about twelve dollars a month. Although the brand name Rogaine is practically synonymous with minoxidil, there are generics that are cheaper.

Although Rogaine is sold in blue boxes for men and pink boxes for women, the drug is exactly the same in both; only the lengths of the applicators are different for different lengths of hair. The manufacturers of Rogaine also make a shampoo called Progaine, but don't waste your money on this, since there is no evidence that it is any better than any other shampoo. Any shampoo that claims to help hair grow is a gimmick.

Hair removal

Needless to say, it is much easier to remove hair than to grow it. Men, who have the greatest experience in removing unwanted hair—most perform the ritual daily—have mostly come to the conclusion that shaving is best.

Many women feel this way too, at least as far as the hair on their legs and underarms is concerned, but when it comes to their faces, they are more inclined to use chemicals, since shaving is perceived as a male thing. There are also still some people who believe that shaving increases hair growth, thickness, and darkness. But this is a myth, for neither shaving nor anything else you do to the external shaft of a hair can influence the way it grows.

The OTC products for hair removal include waxes and chemical depilatories. Waxes, which are often used in salons, are applied to the affected area, allowed to harden, then stripped off. This is the same as pulling out all the hair at once. Chemical products that contain barium sulfide (such as Magic Shave) actually dissolve the hair protein. Along with dissolving the hair protein, they also dissolve some of the skin protein, and the result is that irritation is frequent.

As a cosmetic alternative, dark hair can be bleached so that it is not so noticeable. Electrolysis is also an alternative, and is usually performed by practitioners with a state license. It is the only method of permanent hair removal. An electrical current is used to destroy the root of the hair. Lasers are the newest hair removal devices, but it is too early to determine how well they work and how safe they are.

If you are a woman who has noticed recent increased hair growth, particularly if it is associated with symptoms such as acne, deepening of your voice, weight gain, or irregular menstrual periods, you need a diagnostic workup for endocrine abnormalities. Even if there is nothing detected, hormonal and other drug therapy can be given to reduce unwanted hair when it is very unsightly.

Insect bites

Most biting or stinging insects produce two types of reaction, one that occurs immediately and another that is delayed for about a day. The immediate reaction is a hive, or wheal, which is a red itchy bump that goes away in minutes or hours. The delayed reaction is a firmer, smaller, but more persistent red itchy bump that can last for days. Sometimes, the delayed reaction is a blister.

The types of reaction vary greatly among individuals. Two people can be bitten at the same time by the same bugs, one of them getting a severe reaction and the other showing no ill effects whatsoever. At the extremes, some people may deny being bitten at all, while others are so sensitive that they go into shock and die.

Although there are many hundreds of problem insects, the most common ones are mosquitoes, flies, fleas, ticks, bedbugs, and stinging insects.

Mosquitoes are found around the world. Although usually only annoying, they are capable of transmitting serious diseases, such as malaria, yellow fever, and encephalitis. Only the females bite. They are attracted by moisture (sweat), carbon dioxide (in exhaled breath), warmth, and bright colors.

Flies, such as horseflies, deer flies, black flies, sand flies, and gnats, can cause a variety of problems, depending upon their size and their tendency to swarm.

Fleas, which primarily affect dogs and cats, will sometimes jump up from the ground if their preferred host is not available and cause bites that tend to be worst from the knees down. In some parts of the world fleas transmit plague and other diseases.

Ticks are bloodsucking insects that transmit Lyme disease, Rocky Mountain spotted fever, and other diseases. There are many types. Some feed on specific species, while others attack anything that moves. They are found primarily in woody or grassy areas.

Bedbugs are found in all sections of society, from rich to poor, and usually don't wake you up when they bite. The symptom of their presence is likely to be bloody sheets or bedclothes caused by scratching during the night. They hide, not only in mattresses and other furniture, but also in the cracks between the walls and the floor.

Stinging insects such as bees, wasps, and fire ants can cause very painful bites and stings and are responsible for a surprising number of deaths every year from allergic reactions.

Mild insect bites can be treated by local application of an ice cube and **hydrocortisone** cream, whereas the severe ones need prompt medical treatment with injected **epinepherine**. If bites become infected they need prescription antibiotics.

Numerous other products similar to those available for poison ivy and sunburn are available for local treatment, including local anesthetics such as **benzocaine, dibucaine,** and **lidocaine,** topical antihistamines such as **diphenhydramine** and **tripelennamine,** and calamine (**zinc oxide**), **menthol,** and **camphor.** Unfortunately, they only act for a very short period of time. Furthermore, **benzocaine** and **diphenhydramine** sometimes cause more irritation than they relieve.

Obviously it is better to prevent bites than treat them. Wearing enough clothes to cover exposed skin is a good idea and in extreme cases nets and masks may be necessary. **DEET** has been the most effective insect repellent for many years and is the one present in almost all commercially available products, such as Off! and Repel. Its range of effectiveness, however, is not great and it only reaches about an inch and a half in each direction, so that it must be applied strategically. It is generally safe for most fabrics but can damage some synthetics, such as rayon, and plastics.

DEET comes in a range of strengths; the lower concentrations are for children and the higher concentrations are for maximum protection. But it is doubtful whether concentrations above about fifty percent protect enough more to make them worthwhile. Concentrations above that level may last a little longer, but are not necessarily better.

Permethrin is a better repellent than **DEET** for ticks and has the advantage of also being an insecticide. It can be sprayed on clothing and tents.

Avon Skin So Soft has a reputation as an effective insect repellent, probably because it contains a small amount of **oil of citronella.** If for some reason you prefer **oil of citronella,** however, there are products that contain it in higher concentration.

Itching

Itching, like pain, is a sensation we have all experienced at one time or another. Also like pain, it is not a disease but a symptom of a disease. Medically it can be divided into two types, itching in which some rash or other visible abnormality is present, and itching in which the skin appears normal.

A rash is helpful because it provides clues to the nature of the problem. But many conditions cause itching, such as hives, insect bites, allergies, eczema, ringworm, prickly heat, chickenpox, lice, poison ivy, and bacterial skin infections, to name a very few.

If you can identify the rash, obviously you should treat it specifically. Clearing it up will clear up the itching. Unfortunately, this is often not possible without an outside expert opinion, and one is left with the problem of treating a symptom without knowing what is causing it.

Although most causes of generalized itching are not serious, kidney disease, liver disease, diabetes, intestinal parasites, and even cancer can produce severe, chronic itching, with or without a rash.

There are a few things one should know about itching:

- Itching that is generalized or that hops from one area of the body to another and occurs in the fall or winter is often the type of eczema called winter itch and is mainly caused by dry skin. Many people with dry skin don't appreciate how much itching it can cause.
- Itching that wakes you up at night may be due to scabies, a mite infestation. This needs a *prescription* form of **permethrin**.
- Itching that is localized to one or two areas that you constantly rub, dig, and scratch and that looks leathery is very likely a form of chronic eczema.

There are several external and internal OTC products that act nonspecifically to help reduce itching and should be considered for temporary use only. If the itching subsides completely and quickly, all is well, but if these products don't work you need medical attention.

External anti-itch ingredients consist of the following

ingredients, either alone or in combination: **benzocaine, dibucaine, pramoxine, diphenhydramine, tripelennamine, phenol, camphor, benzyl alchol, menthol, oatmeal, lidocaine,** and **methyl salicylate. Hydrocortisone** is also labelled for itching, but is in a category by itself.

There are several problems with these ingredients. The first is that they do not work very well or very long. The second is that they may cause allergies, rashes, and itching by themselves, thereby compounding the problem. This is most notable with the anesthetic **benzocaine** and the antihistamine **diphenhydramine.** The third problem is that they are not specific and usually do nothing for the underlying condition.

If you want to try an external product, one of the **pramoxine** products, such as Anti-Itch or Caladryl, can be used for a short period of time. If it doesn't work, the others are not likely to be any better.

Internal anti-itch products are the antihistamines, such as **diphenhydramine** (Benadryl). Allergies to **diphenhydramine** taken internally are very uncommon, which is not the case when it is applied to the skin. Antihistamines are most effective when taken at night. During the day they cause too much sedation.

In general, if you are tempted to buy something OTC for itching, your first and last question should be: Itching from what? If you know the answer, treat it appropriately. If you don't, find someone who does.

Jock itch

As its name implies, this disease causes redness, itching, or burning of the upper inner thighs and groin area. It is far more common in men than women.

The skin in this location is delicate and tends to get hot, and perspiration, tight underwear, and the rubbing of skin on skin, especially in those who are overweight or muscular, can cause jock itch, which is sometimes nothing more than irritation or chafing from friction. If we were animals in the jungle and felt discomfort between our legs we would probably raise our tails, spread our legs, and let everything air out for a while, but as responsible members of society with jobs and reputations to uphold we can't do that.

Sometimes infection with true funguses and yeasts occurs in the groin area. The ringworm fungus, which also causes athlete's foot, looks like a ring—the margin is redder, more scaly, sharper, and more elevated than the center. A yeast, on the other hand, is more diffusely red and raw, often having red bumps or pimples that extend beyond the margin of the rash.

Nine times out of ten, a man who has ringworm jock itch also has ringworm athlete's foot. The infection is transferred from feet to groin when he pulls on his underwear. And nine times out of ten, a woman who has ringworm jock itch (which is rare) has a sexual partner with a fungus infection of a hand.

Although the same ingredients used to treat ringworm and athlete's foot can be used for jock itch, only products that contain either **clotrimazole** or **miconazole** should be considered in view of the tendency for the groin to become irritated. These ingredients are interchangeable and are found in the Lotrimin and Micatin product lines, among others. Another advantage of these two ingredients is that they also kill yeasts. It is not always easy to tell a yeast infection from a true ringworm fungus infection of the groin, so if you don't know exactly what's going on, the shotgun approach to treatment is more effective.

If you still have a groin irritation after two weeks of faithful topical treatment with a ringworm medication, it almost certainly isn't being caused by a germ. The problem could be a frictional type of jock itch, or your own rubbing and scratching may be keeping the area inflamed. In this case, the condition is a type of eczema; try **hydrocortisone** in a cream form (as opposed to an ointment, or greasy form).

Lice

Lice come in three varieties: head lice, pubic lice, and body lice.

Head lice cause itching of the scalp, most commonly in children. The insects, though tiny, can be seen with the naked eye, as can their eggs (nits), which appear as white dots cemented firmly to the hair filament.

Teachers and nurses are usually the first to notice an outbreak at a school and often inform parents of the problem by form letter. If you receive such a letter there is no need to be alarmed; head lice are found in expensive private schools as well as public schools. You don't need to see a doctor if the diagnosis is correct because OTC products work at least as well as just about anything available by prescription.

Two related ingredients are used in all of these products, **pyrethrins,** which are derived from a type of chrysanthemum, and **permethrin,** which is a related synthetic compound. The **pyrethrins** are combined with another chemical, **piperonyl butoxide,** which helps them work. The **permethrin** products are generally more effective, because they kill the eggs as well as living insects. The **pyrethrin-piperonyl butoxide** products do not kill nits, so treatment must often be repeated.

There are various types of rinses, shampoos, gels, and liquids that are designed to be applied to the infested area and left in place for ten minutes. They are then rinsed out with warm water. They are usually well tolerated but skin irritation can develop. Mild and temporary stinging or itching is fairly common and is nothing to be concerned about, but you should avoid overusing these products. The belief that if ten minutes is good, twenty might be better is not true here and following it may cause irritation. Many of these products are sold with fine-toothed combs for nit removal, but these are not essential.

Some strains of head lice seem to have developed a resistance to these insecticides and occasional cases can be extremely stubborn. There is even talk of a strain of a super louse that is evolving. If you seem to be fighting a losing battle with lice, having gone through several retreatments, you may have to resort to a messy but effective alternative: coat the infested hair with a generous amount of plain **petrolatum** (petroleum jelly) and leave it on overnight, sleeping in a shower cap. It may take a week or more of daily shampooing to get out the goo, but the lice will have suffocated.

Pubic lice, which attach themselves to the pubic hair, are a different species of insect. Because they look like tiny crabs under a microscope they are called crab lice, and the disease they cause is called crabs. It is a sexually transmitted disease that causes intense itching in the pubic area. Although the same medications used for head lice work also for pubic lice, the FDA does not include pubic lice in the approved indications.

The situation with body lice is different. Whereas head and pubic lice live in hair, body lice live in the seams of unwashed clothing. Normal laundering and good hygiene will get rid of them.

Nails

Fingernails

Despite the belief that general health and nutritional status are important to the way your fingernails look, most nail trouble is from external wear and tear. Splitting, thinning, and failure to grow are almost always caused by small but repetitive daily injuries: certain occupations and hobbies, as well as housework, take their toll on fingernails and you tend to deposit a little nail tissue here and there throughout your environment. Sometimes, cosmetic treatments just make it worse. Buffing the nails to make them smooth, for instance, can make them thin and even more fragile. Contrary to popular opinion, neither gelatin or calcium supplements will strengthen nails.

There are two common fingernail problems that can be treated OTC. The first is separation of the nail itself from the underlying skin. This usually starts at the tip of the nail and extends backwards. There may be a green or greenish black discoloration of the nail.

This condition (called onycholysis) is most often caused by infection by a germ that burrows under the nail. The germ manufactures an enzyme that helps the tissue separate, and cleaning out debris from beneath the nail—particularly the greenish discoloration—will push the infection further back. Treatment is to clip your nail(s) back as far as you comfortably can and soak them in a solution of plain white vinegar and water, fifty-fifty. Do this for five to ten minutes two times a day for a month and then see if the nail grows out normally.

The other condition is a redness and puffiness of the skin around the nail. This is called paronychia.

Paronychia that occurs suddenly, with swelling and significant pain, is most likely bacterial and needs a prescription antibiotic, but longstanding paronychia, with several fingers involved, is most likely a combination of inflammation and a yeast infection. Equal parts of a one-percent **hydrocortisone** cream mixed with a **miconazole** or **clotrimazole** cream applied two times a day may prove helpful. This treatment may need to be continued for many weeks or months.

This kind of inflammation is made worse if the cuticle is not present. Cuticles should never be cut or pushed back; they are important in maintaining a seal between the nail itself and the skin around it.

Toenails

Most toenail trouble falls into one of two categories: fungus infections and ingrown toenails.

Ringworm fungus makes nails thick, yellow, distorted, and crumbly. It is associated with athlete's foot and only a prescription oral medication will get rid of it.

Although there is no FDA approved ingredient for ingrown toenails, this doesn't mean you can't do anything about them. Furthermore, if you understand how they develop, you should never get one.

It used to be thought that ingrown toenails were caused by how you cut your nails. This is not true. Ingrown nails are due entirely to wearing shoes that are too tight for your feet and that pinch your toes together. It is almost always the great toes that are affected. Not wearing shoes, or wearing the widest ones you can, will both prevent and treat the problem. You can trim your nails any way you want: straight across or with a curve.

Every so often, however, the problem is so acute that a small surgical procedure is called for. This involves cutting out the offending nail under local anesthesia, then allowing the nail to regrow without the tight shoes that caused the problem to begin with.

The formerly available OTC products for ingrown nails have been taken off the market. Those whose names might lead you to believe in their effectiveness usually contain local anesthetics such as **benzocaine,** but they are of very limited value and cannot be recommended.

Pigmentation problems

Disturbances in skin color are either those where the skin is darker than normal or those where it is lighter than normal.

Dark spots

Freckles, the mask of pregnancy (called melasma), and moles (beauty marks) all cause dark spots or patches. People with dark or black skin are very prone to increased pigmentation after cuts, scrapes, burns, skin infections, or acne pimples.

Unfortunately, another cause of dark spots is the skin cancer known as melanoma. Since this potentially deadly cancer can be so difficult to diagnose it is wise to have any unusual pigmented lesion looked at by an expert. Only if you are certain that it's nothing to worry about should you consider treating it yourself. But then your decision is easy, because despite the variety of commercial products sold, there is only one active ingredient, **hydroquinone.**

This chemical is not a bleach in the common sense, and how it works isn't exactly known, although it has something to do with interfering with the manufacture of melanin, the substance that gives skin its color. Unfortunately, **hydroquinone** is not too effective, and some people develop an irritation from it. The two-percent concentration is available OTC, whereas higher strengths, up to four percent, can be obtained by prescription.

You should apply the **hydroquinone** product twice a day for three months or so. If it hasn't worked by then it isn't likely to. Don't forget to wear a sunblock during this time, because even a little ultraviolet light tends to darken blotchy skin considerably.

Light spots

Patches of light skin, which are secondary to vitiligo (Michael Jackson's disease), injuries, or congenital absence of pigment, cannot be treated with any OTC product. There are two other conditions, however, in which the skin loses pigment as a secondary phenomenon which can be self treated.

156

The first is a type of fungus infection that usually occurs on the chest or back, gets worse every summer, and shows up as splotches of light skin that have a sharply defined edge and very slight scale. The medical term for this is tinea versicolor and it is commonly called sun fungus. One of the ringworm creams such as **clotrimazole** or **miconazole** used two times a day for two weeks will usually clear it up, although you may have to use it every year when the condition recurs.

The second condition is a type of eczema that usually shows up on the cheeks or upper arms as splotches of white skin with an *indistinct* edge (as opposed to the sharp edge of the fungus condition). Children with eczema and dark skin are particularly prone to this. A one-percent **hydrocortisone** ointment (greasy form) should help this.

Pinworms

Although the very thought of worms wiggling in and out of one's rectum is enough to give most people nightmares, it is important to consider an infestation of pinworms as a cause of anal itching, sleeplessness, and irritability, particularly in children.

Although the worms live within the intestines, the females crawl out at night to deposit their eggs around the anus, which causes itching. The victim then scratches and gets some eggs on his or her fingers. Since the eggs are sticky and survive for weeks, they can be deposited on household utensils or doorknobs. From here, they can be transferred to other people or to food. Once the eggs are eaten, the cycle can start again. Entire families and people in all walks of life can be infested.

The simplest, cheapest, and quickest way to discover if a child is infested is by direct examination. A responsible family member should sneak into the child's room an hour or so after he or she has gone to bed. A small flashlight can then used to examine the anal area. If the worms are present, they will be seen crawling about.

Another way to test for pinworms is to use the Scotch Tape test. Commercial kits with instructions are available, but the basic method is to attach one end of a piece of clear tape to a glass slide. Again, a responsible family member is designated to collect the specimen at night. The tape is rolled back, sticky side out, and pressed against the skin around the anus four times, once in each quadrant. The free end of the tape is then fastened to the other side of the glass slide and transported to the laboratory, where it is examined under a microscope for worms or eggs. A positive test proves infestation with pinworms, but a negative test does not rule it out.

The treatment for pinworms is available OTC. In fact, it is the only intestinal worm you can treat yourself. The active ingredient, **pyrantel pamoate,** is identical in all preparations, so buy the least expensive product you can find and follow the manufacturer's recommendations.

All family members should be treated, even those without symptoms, because some may be carriers and not know it. All sheets, bed linens, night garments, underwear, and towels should be washed simultaneously. Ordinary laundry detergent and warm water is enough. In addition, clip everyone's nails short, have them wash their hands before meals, and institute a program of morning showers or baths, paying particular attention to the anal area, to remove eggs that may have been deposited during the night.

Poison Ivy

The rash from poison ivy is a good example of what is called contact dermatitis, in which a rash results from physically coming in contact with a chemical or other irritating substance.

There are two types of contact dermatitis. The first is a true allergy; the rash does not develop in everyone, only in those allergic to the substance in question. The second type is due to simple irritation and will occur in anyone exposed to a sufficient amount or concentration of the chemical. Poison ivy is an example of the first type, although well over ninety percent of all people are allergic to it.

The rashes from poison ivy, poison oak, and poison sumac look exactly the same; the only way you can tell them apart is by examining the plants themselves. The rash appears one to three days after exposure and is usually streaky looking, appearing as bumps and blisters in lines.

When severe, the blisters can become enormous and exude large amounts of fluid.

There are a few points about poison ivy contact dermatitis that are important to keep in mind:

- If you wash the resin (oil) off your skin within five minutes of touching it, you won't get the rash.
- You can't spread poison ivy once you have the rash, either to yourself or to others. The fluid that comes from the blisters will not cause the eruption to spread.
- Clothing, gardening gloves, gardening tools, or pets may harbor the resin and contribute to the eruption.
- It is very uncomfortable but not dangerous.

The best you can hope for with any type of OTC treatment is temporary relief; you can't shorten the duration of the rash, which can last two to three weeks. If the eruption is very mild and not weeping, use one of the **hydrocortisone** creams three or four times a day. To help you sleep at night take an oral antihistamine such as **diphenhydramine.**

If there are blisters leaking fluid, compresses with an astringent such as **aluminum acetate** are useful. Astringents dry up these fluids better than plain tap water. When the leaking stops, usually after a few days, you can apply the **hydrocortisone** cream.

Although approved for use in poison ivy, local anesthetics such as **benzocaine** and *externally* applied antihistamines such as **diphenhydramine** are best avoided since the relief they provide is very temporary and it is possible to develop additional allergies to them.

If the rash is even moderately severe or uncomfortable, it is best to see a doctor. A stronger, prescription-strength steroid cream such as clobetasol (Temovate and generics) or a short course of a prescription steroid such as prednisone are very effective at alleviating symptoms.

Because it is hard to treat yourself adequately for poison ivy, it is better to prevent it. For this, you want to know what the various toxic plants look like. This is not always easy, since poison ivy itself can grow as as vine or a shrub in various forms. Furthermore, there are several varieties of sumac, many of which are not toxic. If you spend a lot of time outdoors, it would be in your best interest to familiarize yourself with the different varieties.

Clothing and gloves are very helpful when working in the garden or when hiking in the woods, but you have to make sure that you don't touch the outside of the fabric, since it can soak up some of the resin.

A protective product containing **bentoquatam** is available and is applied in a thick layer to form a clay-like covering on the skin. It is not known whether it acts as a simple barrier or actually combines with the resin, but it seems to prevent plant dermatitis about seventy percent of the time. Some other barrier creams are available but tend to be messy. One, called Stokogard, leaves an oily residue on the skin that doesn't feel good. Some workers, such as telephone linemen, cannot avoid toxic plants and might find these products useful. If you work outdoors you might ask your employer to cover the cost of a trial run.

Ringworm

Most people know or strongly suspect they have typical ringworm because of its appearance: it is a rash with a red scaly circle in the shape of a ring. It is not a worm but a fungus (mold) which can affect skin, hair, and nails. Ringworm may be contracted from other humans, from animals, or from the soil. There are many different species of these germs.

Children are particularly prone to ringworm, especially on the scalp, and many schools continue to have epidemics. In this form the rash may not look at all like a ring and may be hard to diagnose. Anything that looks like dandruff, especially if it is associated with patchy loss of hair, should be checked by a doctor, since external OTC medications aren't effective enough to treat scalp ringworm.

High-school wrestlers also have a high incidence of ringworm from their close physical contact and frequent abrasion of the skin. Many times the proper medication is used but repeated exposure renews the infection.

Although there are several OTC ringworm medications,

clotrimazole and **miconazole** are the best. They are equally effective and should work within four weeks if applied faithfully two times a day. Not every rash in the shape of a ring is ringworm, of course. It is most likely to be confused with a type of eczema that has a tendency to show up in round patches. The skin eruption of Lyme disease is also circular. If your ringworm symptoms are not gone in a month of treatment, you need to reevaluate the situation.

Skin infections with bacteria

Bacteria such as *Staphylococcus* or *Streptococcus* can produce a number of different problems when they colonize the skin:

- *Impetigo* is a superficial infection that starts as a red spot, develops into a fragile blister, and dries to form a crust the color of honey.
- *Folliculitis* consist of red bumps, with or without a dot of pus, that occur in the hair follicle. Acne is actually a form of folliculitis.
- *Boils* and *abscesses* (furuncles and carbuncles) are deep infections that often need to be drained of their pus.

OTC antibiotics, which are all topical, should *not* be used to treat any of these conditions. The reason for this is that although *very* mild cases of superficial infections (such as impetigo) might respond to them, it is far better to use a prescription antibiotic to clear the problem up effectively and to prevent complications. Treating a boil, for example, with an antibiotic ointment is useless: the antibiotic cannot possibly penetrate through the skin enough to work. Similarly, a product such as Boil Ease, which contains **benzocaine** and **phenol,** will provide temporary relief at best and will delay proper treatment.

For the most part, therefore, OTC antibiotic ointments such as **bacitracin, neomycin,** or **polymyxin B** (see Chapter 14 on first aid) are only useful in preventing infections in clean wounds, not for treating them.

Soaps

Pure soap, a mixture of lye and fat, is actually quite harsh and irritating when used repeatedly for washing. Ivory bar soap, for instance, although a very pure soap and a very good cleanser, can be hard on those with sensitive skin or eczema. Soaps with antiseptics, germicides, or fragrances can also cause skin irritation, particularly in the winter, when they are often used during long, hot showers or baths.

Many dermatologists recommend the use of Dove because of an old study that showed it to be the mildest among several detergents that were tested. Other bar cleansers, such as Alpha Keri, Aveeno, Basis, Camay, Cetaphil, Eucerin, Oil of Olay, Oilatum, and Neutrogena, claim to be good for dry and sensitive skin, but there is little to recommend one over the other except price. Trial and error is the best way to decide which is best for you. For those who can't seem to tolerate soap and water in any form, Cetaphil lotion or something similar can be used as a skin cleanser.

Sunburn

Both depth and the total area involved are taken into consideration in assessing sunburn severity. Certain drugs (photosensitizers) may increase your susceptibility to sunburn. Among these are some antibiotics, antidepressants, birth control pills, blood pressure medications, and analgesics. Read printed information or the package insert or refer to the Physician's Desk Reference and take extra care when taking any medication if you are going to be out of doors. Appendix VI provides a list of OTC products that may cause photosensitivity. Be careful also when applying sunscreens, since burns often occur in the spots you miss.

If the burn is uncomfortable, taking an internal analgesic such as **aspirin, ibuprofen, ketoprofen,** or **naproxen** (see Chapter 22 on pain) will be helpful. Take the full dose regularly; don't wait for the pain to appear. An ointment containing one of the FDA approved protectants, such as **petrolatum, allantoin, cocoa butter,** or **shark liver oil,** may be applied to prevent the sore spots from rubbing against clothing and sheets. **Petrolatum** (petroleum jelly) is as good as any and is very inexpensive. If the area is small and the skin is *unbroken,* **hydrocortisone** cream or ointment may be used three to four times a day. The ointment (greasy) form, although messy, will provide more comfort than the cream. Cool compresses with plain tap water will soothe smaller burns but should be avoided if the area is large. If the skin is broken, see a doctor.

Although approved for use in sunburns, the local anesthetics **benzocaine, lidocaine, dibucaine, benzyl alcohol, butamben,** and **pramoxine** provide only limited value. This is because their effects only last for at most an hour and they should definitely not be used more than three or four times a day. At the very best, therefore, you will only get four hours of relief a day. Furthermore, local anesthetics cause allergic skin irritation in some people.

Prevention, of course, should be the goal. Besides being painful and difficult to treat, sunburn causes melanoma, one of the deadliest forms of cancer.

Sunscreens

Sunscreens remain a great source of confusion to the public, to the medical profession, and to the FDA itself, even though the matter has been simplified somewhat with the introduction of the SPF (Sun Protective Factor), a number by which sunscreens with different compositions can be compared.

In order to understand what's going on, you have to understand something about SPFs, and for that you need a little arithmatic. Let's say that you have fair skin and you might normally get sunburned after twenty minutes of sun exposure on a certain day. Applying an SPF 6 sunscreen means that you'd need two hours of sun (twenty minutes times six) on that day to get an equivalent sunburn. An SPF 15 would allow you to stay out for five hours (twenty minutes times fifteen).

Critics of sunscreens point out that it's not so simple. The SPF refers to a particular bandwidth of ultraviolet light, called ultraviolet B (UVB), which causes sunburn. There is another type, ultraviolet A (UVA), which also damages the skin, and which many sunscreens do not protect against. Nor is it easy to measure exactly how much protection against UVA a particular sunscreen affords.

The main problem with the entire subject is that the disease we are trying to prevent, skin cancer, takes decades to develop, and decades have not yet elapsed since the onset of widespread sunscreen use. One argument against sunscreens is that they actually encourage one to stay out in the sun for abnormally long periods of time, thereby allowing enormous amounts of UVA to hit the skin, a situation whose repercussions will only be known with time. Another argument against them is that many people have a false sense of security and in general do not apply enough sunscreen. Statistics show that this is true.

Both of these situations, however, are easy to avoid by making sure you apply enough sunscreen and by not baking yourself for hours at the beach. When used correctly, sunscreens can save your skin and potentially save your life. The only problem left to solve is deciding which one, of the over one hundred twenty available sunscreens, is best.

One way to discuss the ingredients is to divide them into two groups: those that absorb light and those that block light. Because those that absorb light are transparent, they are much more cosmetically acceptable, and so there are more of them.

The following nine absorbing sunscreen ingredients are available: **avobenzone, homosalate, padimate O, menthyl anthranilate, octocrylene, octyl methoxycinnamate, octyl salicylate, oxybenzone,** and **phenylbenzimidazole sulfonic acid.**

There are two blocking sunscreens: **titanium dioxide** and **zinc oxide.**

Except for a few exceptions, most of these ingredients are found in various combinations of two, three, or four together in order to take advantage of their individual good qualities, such as the ability to stick to the skin well, to resist water, and to provide a broad range of ultraviolet protection.

Table 12. Skin types and recommended sunscreens

Skin type	Description	SPF
I	always burns easily, never tans	30
II	always burns easily, tans a little	20
III	sometimes burns, tans slowly	15
IV	sometimes burns a little, tans well	8
V	rarely burns, tans very well	4

If you're an average adult you need about an ounce of sunscreen to cover yourself, and you need to make a conscious effort not to miss any spots. Apply sunscreens about thirty minutes *before* going outside and reapply as necessary.

Sunscreens, when used properly, tend to cause little trouble, but they may irritate the skin or produce pimples (folliculitis) in some people. If this happens, try one of the products designed for children. They are a bit more expensive, but they are formulated to be gentler. Most of the time it isn't the active ingredient itself that causes the trouble but rather things like perfumes, preservatives, or alcohol.

There really is no practical way to choose a sunscreen other than by relying upon the accuracy of a label for SPF values, water resistance, and spectrum of coverage. There is no ideal list of ingredients. Problems with sensitivity tend to develop as new sunscreen chemicals are introduced into various brand name products; the formulations often change. As far as the FDA is concerned, this topic is in flux. The FDA has published a tentative final monograph on sunscreens and it is still deliberating over the final monograph, a process that usually takes years.

The recommendations in Table 12 for which SPF is best for your skin type are higher than those usually recommended for a simple reason: it's better to be obsessive about protection. Furthermore, if there is a history of skin cancer in your family, use a 30 SPF sunscreen no matter what your skin type is. Try to get a product that covers both UVA and UVB and that is labelled waterproof or very water resistant. Once you have selected a product that meets these conditions, obtain the cheapest one and give it a try. If it feels good and doesn't cause trouble, buy it in bulk.

Warts, corns, and calluses

Although it is not always easy to tell warts, corns, and calluses apart, every effort should be made to do so, since the right treatment is quite different for each.

A wart is caused by a local skin infection with a virus. You usually catch the virus by being scraped or scratched by some object that has virus particles on it, such as a fingernail or sharp object. Because the incubation period is somewhere between two and six months—the period of time during which the infection is invisible, though present—it is next to impossible to trace exactly where you contracted the virus. Nor is it important, except to avoid further infections.

How can you tell if something is a wart? The surface is almost always rough and there are often tiny black dots within it. Although the black dots are sometimes called seeds, they are actually minute blood vessels that contain clotted blood. There is no such thing as a seed wart.

The following points should be noted about warts:

- Some people are much more prone to them than other people, and probably nobody is completely immune. Children get more of them than adults.
- The infection with the virus is local to the skin; it is not in your bloodstream.
- By definition, any wart on the sole of the foot is called a plantar wart. The problem with a plantar wart is that if it is on a weight bearing zone it will be pushed up and deeper into your skin as you walk.
- There are many different varieties of wart (papilloma) virus and each has its own peculiarities, growth requirements, and lifespan.
- Warts will almost always—over ninety-nine percent of the time—go away on their own, but it can take five years for an individual wart to resolve.
- One common wart variant is called a molluscum. Children in particular may develop hundreds of them. They look a bit like tiny volcanoes, small bumps with a tiny crater in the center.

- Common viral warts do not lead to skin cancer, although some skin cancers are warty in appearance.

There is only one OTC FDA approved ingredient for wart removal, **salicylic acid**. It comes in two strengths, a seventeen-percent liquid or gel, and a forty-percent patch, plaster, or adhesive strip. You should try the weaker strength first unless you have a plantar wart, in which case you should go with the stronger. Buy the cheapest product, since they are all identical. When applied correctly, **salicylic acid** will turn the wart and the surrounding skin white. This dead tissue should be removed when it gets loose enough, which is usually after a few days. If the wart remains the process can be repeated.

If the wart isn't gone within a reasonable time—three months is about right—and you don't want to wait for it to spontaneously resolve, you'll have to see a doctor, who will most likely freeze it with liquid nitrogen or burn it with electric current. Laser treatment is indicated only rarely. The success rate for treating some warts isn't good, no matter what *anyone* uses. Some of them go away easily and quickly, whereas others are much more stubborn.

There are two types of growth on the sole of the foot that can be confused with warts: corns and calluses. Both of these are due to pressure and constant rubbing, not infection. Unlike warts, calluses and corns will often be symmetrical, one or more on each foot in a mirror image. Favorite sites for them are on the outside of the little toes, between the little toe and fourth toe, and in the mid portion of the sole about where the toes meet the foot itself (metatarsal heads).

A corn is just a callus that has gotten out of control. The buildup of tissue acts as a foreign body, which causes even more buildup of tissue, so that a painful mass results. Corns on the little toes are from wearing shoes that are too tight and they will go away with the proper footwear. Corns on the soles of the feet may be caused by pressure from bones within your foot. The problem often gets worse as we age, since we lose fat from the bottoms of our feet. If you have corns, buy the softest, roomiest, most cushiony shoes you can find and see if that helps. A doughnut-shaped corn pad may also provide some comfort. If these measures don't work you'll need to see a doctor. Paring down the excess tissue with a razor blade is potentially dangerous.

Calluses are a natural response of the body to repeated trauma and are a protective device. If you didn't have a callus you might very well have a blister. Unless they are painful there is no need to remove them. If you feel they are unsightly, a pumice stone can be used to file them down a little.

Wrinkles

Nowadays, anti-wrinkle creams include one of two main ingredients: sunscreens and alpha hydroxy acids (AHAs).

Theoretically, sunscreens work because too much ultraviolet light makes you look older. But sunscreens only prevent new wrinkles from forming and do nothing for those already there. (See above for more about sunscreens.)

AHAs, on the other hand, may help your appearance, although the improvement won't be dramatic. Since their introduction, AHAs have quickly become the most popular ingredient in various heavily advertised "miracle" creams. Part of their appeal lies in their being natural fruit acids. The most prevalent AHAs are **glycolic acid** and **lactic acid**. There is no evidence that either one is more effective or safer than the other and they can be considered to be interchangeable.

Externally applied AHAs give skin an unusual irritated feeling; when they are first applied they often sting and redden the skin. This effect is transient and does not mean that irritation is more likely to develop with continued use. This temporary effect, however, is psychologically powerful, and the general and immediate sense of users is that the chemicals *must* be doing something.

What that something is, however, nobody seems to know for sure. AHAs are not moisturizers per se, although when used with moisturizers they seem to help hydrate the skin. They do increase the rate at which cells divide and they do disrupt the structure of the skin, though. And repeated use can cause significant irritation, especially if strong or highly acidic preparations are used.

Concentrations of ten percent and below are used in OTC

creams. Those above ten percent are used under professional guidance for chemical peels. Although the FDA is still studying the matter, there is evidence that after several months of repeated use people with sun damaged skin who use OTC AHA products will have some visible improvement in skin color and wrinkling. Whether this is only cosmetic, whether it is permanent, and whether it is beneficial over the long term remain to be seen.

One of the buzzwords associated with AHA use is exfoliation, the removal of dead skin cells from the skin. One often assumes that dead skin cells are bad. On the contrary, dead cells form the main protective layer that gives the skin its barrier function. Excessive exfoliation with AHAs will make you more susceptible to the harmful effects of ultraviolet light and will, ironically, actually accelerate aging. The fact is that you really don't have to exfoliate your skin at all; when the cells are dead enough, they fall off by themselves.

If you think you look prematurely old from too much sun, you might be helped to a small degree by an OTC AHA product. If your wrinkles are mainly expression lines, however, AHAs won't do a thing. If the AHAs don't seem to work there are stronger topical drugs available by prescription, such as isotretinoin (Retin-A or Renova) or 5-fluorouracil, that can combat sun damaged skin and precancerous conditions.

You may see advertisements for anti-aging products containing beta hydroxy acids. At first glance this might seem to be an advance over alpha hydroxy acids, but the fact is that this is just a gimmick to describe **salicylic acid**, which is best avoided in wrinkle creams. There is no scientific evidence that it helps, and it can—like alpha hydroxy acids—aggravate the harmful effects of the sun by removing the protective layer of dead cells on the skin's surface.

25

SLEEP AIDS

How and why we sleep is a complex subject, one that is nowhere near fully understood. We know that there are four stages of sleep, and that one of those stages, REM (Rapid Eye Movement) sleep, is very important, and yet we really don't understand why sleep is so essential in the first place. Sleep disturbances are particularly prevalent in the very young and the very old. Babies who sleep through the night are considered remarkable, and the elderly often have fragmented sleep patterns characterized by many episodes of waking and falling back to sleep again.

Everyone has trouble sleeping at one time or another. Usually it is because of something on your mind, an argument with your spouse, or trouble at work. Sleep disturbances of this type, which typically last only a few days, may possibly be helpful by indicating to you the emotional importance of something you may consider minor, and to which you may not be paying sufficient attention.

If you know exactly what's keeping you up, you're probably well on your way to recovery already, even if the problem is continuing. Short-term sleep problems rarely cause serious difficulties. It is when insomnia becomes more chronic that one's health can suffer. One week of constant and unremitting sleeplessness is generally considered to be more than enough to send you to a doctor. Among the many causes of insomnia, depression ranks high on the list. Depression is a very important and insidious disease that can reveal itself in odd and unusual ways, but some form of sleep disturbance is often prominent. It is important to know that depression is also a very treatable disease.

Acute or chronic pain is also a common treatable cause of insomnia. You can treat minor aches and pains yourself (Chapter 22 on pain), but more serious degrees of it need medical attention. In any event, it is crucial to attack the underlying condition rather than the insomnia. Sleeping pills, for example, sometimes actually intensify pain.

Some medical conditions may contribute to the problem of insomnia, especially those that cause you to urinate frequently, such as bladder or prostate diseases, or those that cause breathing difficulties, such as cardiac or respiratory diseases.

Drugs such as **caffeine** and **alcohol** deserve special mention. Everyone knows that coffee will keep you up, but the situation with alcohol is trickier, because it puts many people to sleep, at least initially. After the initial somnolence wears off, however, a period of intensely turbulent sleep can result. Before taking anything for sleep, therefore, decrease or eliminate your intake of other drugs that have psychological effects.

There are two currently available sleep aids to consider, **diphenhydramine** (Sominex and others) and **doxylamine** (Nytol and others). Both are antihistamines. Exactly how they promote sleep is unknown, as are the specifics of how they influence the various sleep cycles, but it is their side effects that make you drowsy. Although they are roughly equivalent, **diphenhydramine** is generally preferred because it has been around longer. Additionally, the generic form is very inexpensive.

Antihistamines are usually very effective, but if taken for more than about a week on consecutive days tolerance can develop, and you won't get the same effect from them. Some individuals, mostly children, have a response opposite to that intended—called idiosyncratic—and the products make them agitated.

Melatonin, the current sleep aid fad, although freely available OTC, is sold as a food supplement and so is exempt from FDA scrutiny. **Melatonin** is a hormone found in the pineal gland, a small structure nestled in the brain. It is produced in response to darkness and is important in regulating sleep and reproductive cycles and in synchronizing these cycles with daily and seasonal fluctuations in light intensity. In polar regions animals have large pineal glands to help deal with the prolonged periods of darkness found there.

There is good evidence that **melatonin** promotes sleep and can be particularly helpful in certain situations. Some blind people with severe sleep disturbances, for example, whose **melatonin** is high during the day and low at night, have shown dramatic improvement with it. There is also evidence that it can be used to reset the sleep cycle and relieve the symptoms of jet lag, although the right dose and the right timing for this is not known.

The main problem with **melatonin** is that not enough is known about it, especially its long-term safety. Although the big draw for it is that it is a naturally occurring hormone, individual hormones in the body are part of an intricate system of hormones that interact with one another. Hormones by definition are potent chemicals that have profound effects in small doses. Administering one hormone always influences another, sometimes with unintended and undesireable results. **Melatonin,** for instance, may increase the level of the hormone prolactin, high levels of which cause the breasts to enlarge and decrease sex drive. In other words, **melatonin** may be good for your sleep life but not for your love life.

The correct dose is also not known, although health food stores sell doses that typically increase blood levels to ten times or more above those normally found during sleep. Such doses keep the blood level high for long periods and can give you a hangover. For these reasons, **melatonin** cannot be recommended.

Valerian cannot be recommended, either. It is an ancient remedy that has been in and out of favor for hundreds of years. It is derived from a plant called *Valeriana officinalis,* which has a wide distribution around the world. Formerly, dried preparations from the root were used to calm agitated (hysterical) patients, the theory being that anyone who could stand to take something that smelled so bad and tasted so awful could learn to control his or her own behavior.

But there is evidence that some substance in the root has

sedative qualities, although the nature of that substance or substances is not exactly known. The main ingredient of valerian is an oil that itself is composed of several different acids. Although touted as a sleep aid and being considered by the FDA, valerian is much too unpredictable and unreliable to use for sleep.

L-tryptophan went through a period of great popularity as a sleep aid, but this faded after a contaminated batch caused many cases of serious illness and a number of deaths. It can also cause a severe reaction when taken with certain antidepressants. You may find health food stores that still push this substance, but don't fall for the pitch.

Recommendations

Try to keep your life on an even keel; those who sleep well are usually those with a clear conscience.

Get into a good sleeping habit: try to go to bed and get up at the same time every day of the week.

Avoid napping during the day. If you cannot avoid them, limit naps to thirty minutes.

Get into a good exercise program, but exercise no closer than three hours to bedtime.

Don't drink, smoke, or take products containing **caffeine** within four hours of bedtime.

Use your bed for sleeping or sex only.

If you tend to wake up in the middle of the night worrying, write down your worries before going to bed. Promise yourself that you will tackle them the next day.

Find something that puts you to sleep, like reading philosophy or watching a black and white movie classic on TV.

Avoid late-night snacks that may give you heartburn.

Make your bed and bedroom nice and cozy, not too hot, cold, bright, or noisy.

If you have a transient sleep disturbance, take one of the **diphenhydramine** preparations.

If you find yourself using an OTC sleep aid for longer than seven consecutive days, see a doctor.

26

STIMULANTS

If you consider coffee, tea, chocolate, and soft drinks as sources of **caffeine**, then this stimulant is by far the most widely used drug in America. The average American adult actually ingests almost two hundred milligrams a day, which means that many are taking in much more. If you are like most people, therefore, the question is not whether or not to take **caffeine** but whether you should be taking more or less of it.

Caffeine, the only FDA approved OTC stimulant, has probably been used for thousands of years, but it is still the subject of intense study, debate, and controversy. Common sense would seem to indicate that it must have some very serious drawbacks as a stimulant.

Over the years attempts have been made to link **caffeine** to high blood pressure, heart disease, fibrocystic disease of the breast, breast cancer, cancer of the pancreas, and cancer of the bladder. For the most part, **caffeine's** relationship to these diseases has never been proven, and they probably have nothing to do with one another. It does appear, however, that **caffeine** consumption in women decreases fertility, and that **caffeine** is associated in an unclear way to high cholesterol, although it remains to be seen whether future research will bear out these findings. Most doctors will tell you to avoid **caffeine** if you suffer heart palpitations or heart rhythm disturbances (arrhythmias), since **caffeine** in high doses definitely affects the heart rate. Although **caffeine** produces a transient rise in blood pressure, it quickly returns to normal, and those with high blood pressure generally do not need to be overly concerned.

Caffeine also increases gastric acidity and is a common cause of heartburn. In general, those with ulcers or digestive problems should avoid it.

The most insidious drawback to **caffeine** is addiction or habituation. Many people *need* their morning cup of coffee, and feel physically and psychologically deprived if they do not have it. Furthermore, even if they realize their dependence, they find it hard to stop. Many of us experience the symptoms of **caffeine** withdrawal every morning as we get ready for work. Weekends may be particularly bad since one's coffee consumption at work is generally higher than at home. Symptoms begin about twelve hours after your last dose and typically include fatigue, depression, and headaches. But **caffeine** is rapidly absorbed into your bloodstream and you will definitely feel much better within half an hour of your pick-me-up.

The effects of **caffeine** are related to the dose. Low or moderate amounts increase energy, alertness, and the ability to concentrate, but as the dose increases, so do side effects, such as nervousness, irritability, shakiness, and insomnia. At high doses, toxicity, known as caffeinism, results, in which side effects are exaggerated. This can be seen after as little as two hundred fifty milligrams, an amount that could be contained in a large mug of strong coffee, although larger amounts, such as one thousand milligrams, more commonly produce the effect. At this point, talkativeness, agitation, muscle twitching, excessive urination, upset stomach, facial flushing, ringing in the ears, and the feeling that one has boundless energy may be seen. As with other drugs that affect the mind, though, tolerance often develops, and some individuals are able to take in fairly large amounts with no apparent ill effects. The lethal dose in humans is estimated to be about 10,000 milligrams (ten grams). Children are much more sensitive to **caffeine** than adults and can get quite a jolt from a single soft drink.

Table 13. Caffeine contents

Food and amount	Caffeine (mg)
brewed coffee (6 oz)	50–150
brewed tea (6 oz)	20–100
colas (12 oz, regular or diet) and Mountain Dew	50
cocoa (6 oz)	2–20
chocolate (1 oz)	1–35

As a point of interest you might add up how much **caffeine** you're taking in right now, especially if you think you're drinking too much coffee or tea or if you suffer from palpitations or frequent headaches, or if you feel depressed late in the afternoon. Think in terms both of your total daily dose and the time of day you are ingesting it. The figures for coffee and tea are highly variable and depend upon how strong they are brewed. Chocolate is also variable, with the dark varieties containing more **caffeine.**

Caffeine pills are manufactured under a number of descriptive and colorful names, such as NoDoz, King of Hearts, Quick-Pep and 357 Magnum II. Most contain 200 milligrams of the ingredient. Do they work? Unquestionably. Within minutes of taking a single dose of any you will feel the kick. But they cannot be recommended. If you're like most people you've got enough **caffeine** on board right now and don't need any more. In fact, you're probably dependent on it. Upset stomach is also far more common with **caffeine** pills than with an equivalent dose of **caffeine** in a natural form.

Recommendations

If you want to cut down on your **caffeine** intake, do it gradually. Calculate how much you're ingesting and reduce it over a week or two, gradually mixing in decaffeinated coffee or tea with your regular brew. Most colas come in decaffeinated varieties.

If you're always fatigued, see a doctor. Anemia and depression are only two of many possible causes of this very common symptom.

27

STOP SMOKING

If you smoke there is nothing better you can do for your health than to quit. Competing with your will power and better judgment is your addiction, one of the strongest forces in the universe. But you can quit, and you should keep trying, no matter how many times you have failed in the past. Most successful quitters make a number of attempts before they are successful.

People start smoking for different reasons. Psychologically, the biggest motivator at first is peer pressure and the desire to appear more adult and sophisticated; smoking still connotes mystery and sex. The initial reaction of most individuals to their first cigarette is to turn green, but one gets over this quickly. Before long, you're hooked.

Dr. C. Everett Koop, former surgeon general, has said that **nicotine** is as addictive as heroin. It is difficult and possibly unfair to make comparisons of this sort, but it is a fact that **nicotine** is one of the strongest and most toxic drugs, with an estimated acute lethal dose of about sixty milligrams, about as much as in half a cigar. As a poison, **nicotine** works as fast as cyanide. The symptoms of **nicotine** poisoning include vomiting, diarrhea, irregularities of the heartbeat, and convulsions.

Nicotine is a chemical with complex effects on the nervous system. It has no known medical value, but is actually valuable as a research tool in probing the intricacies of transmission across synapses—the spaces where nerves meet. In small doses it is a stimulant, whereas in larger doses it affects what is known as the reward center in the brain.

Although **nicotine** is the habituating ingredient in tobacco and is itself harmful, it is the added carbon monoxide, tars, and carcinogens that make smoking the menace that it is. The list of health problems caused or aggravated by smoking include heart disease, high blood pressure, leg cramps, vascular spasms, intestinal problems, lung disease, and cancer. It can also worsen diabetes, thyroid disease, allergies, cataracts, and depression. Cosmetically, it stains teeth, causes bad breath, and induces wrinkles.

Statistics show that most smokers want to quit. Although some people claim that they like to smoke, it is really that they don't like the feelings of anxiety, fear, irritability, panic, craving, and impaired mental capacity they get when they try to stop. Mark Twain summed it up best when he said that quitting was easy: he'd done it thousands of times.

But Twain didn't have modern medicine on his side, and there is good evidence that OTC **nicotine** delivery systems can help a lot in those properly motivated. The key word, however, is *motivated*. Unlike diet pills, which can be taken no matter how much you eat, you have to stop smoking *completely* before you try replacement. This will be your biggest hurdle.

There are two forms of OTC **nicotine**, "chewing gum" and patches (although a third form, a nasal spray now available by prescription, may have changed status by the time you read this). The reason "chewing gum" is in quotes is because it is not ordinary gum nor should it be used as ordinary gum. It is chewed only until it emits a peppery taste—the nicotine—at which point it is parked between the gums and cheek. When the peppery taste leaves you chew a little more for another hit. **Nicotine** is rapidly absorbed from the oral membranes and results can be felt almost at once.

If you decide on the gum you should take it on the recommended schedule, not when you feel that you need it. This will keep your blood **nicotine** at a more stable level and will reduce your discomfort. For this reason you have to carry a supply with you. It comes in two sizes, two and four milligrams, the larger being for those who smoke more than twenty-four cigarettes a day. The schedule consists of one piece of gum every one or two hours for six weeks, then one piece every two to four hours for three weeks, then one piece every four to eight hours for three weeks. You're not supposed to eat or drink for fifteen minutes before using it or while using it. The taste is unusual but not unpleasant.

There are two patch products, Nicoderm CQ and Nicotrol. Nicoderm is designed to be used in a three-step program, going from twenty-one, to fourteen, and then to seven milligrams of **nicotine** a day, whereas Nicotrol comes as a single fifteen-milligram per day dose. The Nicotrol patches are designed to be worn during waking hours only, whereas the Nicoderm patches are worn for twenty-four hours.

The method best for most smokers is probably the graded Nicoderm patch system. The gum is entirely too much of a nuisance, and the different doses of Nicoderm allow one to customize the rate of withdrawal, which should ease the unpleasantness.

The main disadvantage to all of these systems is that they don't raise your blood nicotine level the same way a good drag on a Camel will, and so you may still feel somewhat deprived. Studies do show, however, that you're more likely to quit if you use replacement. If you are successful, of course, you then have to stop the patches, and some people do become addicted to them.

Recommendations

Use the Nicoderm patches and keep trying to quit until you succeed.

Set a target date for quitting. It has been shown that those who prepare themselves psychologically with this date in mind have a better success rate.

Throw away your cigarettes and do everything and anything you can to motivate yourself to stop smoking. Enlist the help of those who love you. Many have found a buddy system helpful, in which a friend encourages you to call if the craving becomes very strong.

If you can't quit completely, try smoking only out of doors, not at home or in your car. Then cut down the sites in which you allow yourself to smoke. Each restriction will get you used to smoking less and will demonstrate that you can not only survive without tobacco, but flourish.

28

URINARY CONDITIONS

Most people are surprised to learn that you can treat yourself for bladder infections (cystitis) at home with OTC products. Whether it is smart to do, obviously, is another matter. The main problem arises because the best way to diagnose these infections, which are properly termed urinary tract infections, or UTIs, is by means of a urine culture, and you can't just go to the laboratory and get a urine culture for yourself without a doctor's order. The best advice, clearly, is not to fool around in this area unless you are under the care of a physician.

Women suffer far more from UTIs than do men because of their anatomy: the urethra, the tube that leads from the bladder to the outside of the body, is much shorter, and consequently, the distance between the bladder and the outside world of contamination is less. Most UTIs arise from such an ascending infection with bacteria. These bacteria are usually the same ones that inhabit the intestine, particularly the colon, which is not surprising given the closeness of the organs of elimination to one another. The bacteria are notoriously resistant to treatment and tend to stay around in some people for a long time.

Another point of anatomy should be stressed here, which is that the bladder and the kidneys are connected by tubes (the ureters). The real danger of these infections is that an actual kidney infection can develop from an infection lower down, and this may lead to kidney failure.

The symptoms of a UTI may include burning, stinging, or pain when you urinate, or the presence of blood in your urine. Fever, nausea, and aches and pains are unusual unless the kidneys are already involved. Some people, however, harbor bacteria in their urine and have no symptoms whatsoever.

There are two OTC ingredients available for these infections: **methenamine** and **phenazopyridine.**

Methenamine is a urinary antiseptic (not an antibiotic) that is over a hundred years old. It is prepared by synthesizing ammonia and formaldehyde; when the compound is excreted in the urine the formaldehyde is released and kills the germs.

Methenamine has two advantages: it is relatively safe and no bacteria have thus far developed a resistance to the formaldehyde. On the negative side, it is somewhat weak as an antiseptic and relies heavily on an acidic urine (pH of about 5, or lower). If your doctor has recommended that you use it, test your urine with one of the urinary testing strips that are available in drug stores. If the pH is above 5, your doctor may recommend taking **ammonium chloride** to acidify your urine.

Phenazopyridine is a urinary analgesic that is meant only to reduce the symptoms of a UTI. If taken for short periods of time in the recommended dose it is relatively safe. It should be kept in mind, however, that **phenazopyridine** should not be used by anyone with diminished kidney function. It also turns the urine an orange color and may interfere with laboratory tests on the urine that rely on color variations.

Although the above drugs are available both in OTC and prescription forms, for the reasons discussed they cannot be recommended for self-treatment.

29

WEIGHT REDUCTION

There is only one currently approved OTC appetite suppressant on the market, **phenylpropanolamine** (PPA). All of the popular brands, including Acutrim, Dexatrim, Permathene, and Protrim, contain it and only it as their active ingredient. Furthermore, they all contain it in the same dose, seventy-five milligrams, in a once-a-day timed release form. You can find other products with less PPA, but the big sellers all contain identical amounts, even those whose labeling might lead you to consider otherwise, such as Acutrim 16 Hour Steady Control, Acutrim Late Day Strength, and Acutrim II Maximum Strength. PPA is related chemically to amphetamines, although the harmful side effects and stimulation are diminished. It is not known exactly how it suppresses appetite, but studies show that it does. It is particularly important not to exceed the recommended doses, however, because PPA can cause very serious side effects if taken in large amounts. It is also important not to take PPA with certain other drugs or medications. Mixing PPA with some heart or psychiatric drugs can be deadly.

In general, PPA is only modestly successful and relies to a great extent upon your own motivation to cut down on your food intake. If you only want to lose a few pounds it is much healthier to do it yourself, without drugs of any kind. As the constant supply of new diet books demonstrates, however, it isn't easy.

Diet

It has been said that nobody actually reads diet books, but buy them to feel virtuous. Losing weight is very hard and it gets harder the older you are. Will power often diminishes with age, as does the ability to exercise; one fatigues faster and is more prone to injury.

The tendency to gain weight is natural. Our ancestors lived through periods of feast and famine, and the survivors were the ones who were able to put on enough fat to live through hard times. We are the descendents of these survivors. Nature is smart in this way, since fat happens to be the most efficient way of storing energy in the body; each gram (1/30 of an ounce) produces about nine calories. On the other hand, this is why fat in one's diet is an enemy: eating just a little bit adds many calories to total dietary intake.

For all the apparent complexity, one's weight is based upon a simple equation:

Weight = Calories in − Calories out

There may be other factors in play, of course. Thyroid or other endocrine diseases can certainly influence weight, but as a rule you can easily find out if you have such a condition. (More than likely, you don't.) Heredity also has a role. Although a number of genes have been identified that control the tendency to put on pounds, there is nothing one can do at this time to change the situation, short of selecting different ancestors.

So you have to concentrate on the calories.

Most experts will tell you to attack the problem on both fronts, by eating less and exercising more, but the fact is that eating less is much more important. The main reason for this is that most adults can't exercise enough to make up for what they're eating. Let's say you average a twenty minute workout every single day, which is just about what most working adults can handle. At a good clip, this will burn up about two hundred calories, again what most people can handle. A few French fries, a candy bar, or a piece of cheesecake will wipe this out in a snap. Moreover, you're actually much more likely to eat those French fries, candy, or cheesecake after exercising, since you feel so virtuous. As experience with diet pills, surgical procedures, and other research has shown, you don't really need to exercise at all to lose a lot of weight; eating less works just fine.

The exception to the above is in children and teenagers. Young people—who are on average now showing a tendency to become heavier (along with the rest of us)—usually become overweight because of a lack of physical activity. They should be encouraged to stick to a nutritious diet and to engage in sports and recreational activities that expend calories. Kids who show sudden changes in weight, by the way, may be showing early signs of depression. Parents should get involved in such cases not only for the health and cosmetic benefits, but also for the youngster's psychological well being.

The importance of restricting calories in adults, however, has nothing to do with the value of exercise for your health. Those who exercise are doing themselves an enormous favor; they just might not lose as much weight as they think they should. The value of eating less is just a matter of what is easier: avoiding the slice of apple pie, or exercising vigorously for the forty-five minutes, more or less, that it takes to burn it off. Most people would choose the former, not because it's easy, just easier. The need for food is like the need for air: you can't ignore your reliance on it.

You might hear the statement that diets don't work. This is simply not true. You will lose weight if you follow them faithfully. However, the habits many of them require cannot be maintained over a long time without superhuman effort. Liquid preparations such as Slim-Fast and Optifast are in this class. If you follow the directions you will definitely lose weight, and quickly. For a time you will have a can of it for breakfast and a can of it for lunch, with a low-calorie dinner, but there inevitably comes the day of reckoning when the bacon and eggs call for breakfast, when the corned beef on rye calls for lunch, or when the chocolate chip cookies call out for dessert after dinner. What do you do then? The habit of drinking chocolate shakes instead of eating two meals a day is impossible to continue over a lifetime, so you quickly gain back the weight you initially lost.

You can find tables of desirable weights in many places. Most are based upon life insurance statistics and are good general guides. The best tables are based upon a figure known as the body mass index, or BMI, and is calculated by dividing one's weight (in kilograms) by the square of one's height (in meters). Although several figures have been proposed as ideal, a BMI of 25 is generally a good number to consider as the upper limit of normal for a given height. Your weight should be below this level. If it is above, you are considered to be overweight.

Another way to use BMIs is as a means to assess relative risk one has of developing diseases because of one's weight. This is detailed in Table 14.

Table 14. Health risks and body mass index (BMI)

BMI	Associated Health Risk
less than 25	Minimal
25–27	Low
27–30	Moderate
30–35	High
35–40	Very high
above 40	Extremely high

The trick to dieting is habit. Overeating is a bad habit; eating right is a good habit. Habits come from repetition. If you keep trying to eat properly, for good health, well being, and nutrition, this will also become a habit.

Eating properly entails controling the volume of food and monitoring its quality.

The advantage to cutting down on the volume is that you can continue to eat what you like. Count up the bon-bons you normally devour at night watching TV and toss away ten percent of them right off the bat. The same goes with the pizza and potato chips. More than likely, you won't feel (overly) deprived. The other advantage to reducing volume by ten percent is that you don't need to know anything at all about the calorie content of food.

Changing the quality of your food means substituting lower calorie foods for higher calorie ones, and for this you need to know something about nutrition. Luckily, the information is freely available. Just looking at a table of calories or at the labels of foods you buy in the supermarket can be an education. The FDA has provided dieters with a great tool by requiring manufacturers to list the calories and fat content of the foods they produce.

If you know how to calculate calories you can fill your stomach and still lose weight.

Every dieter loses will power at some point and gets off track. In some cases this can reach extremes: downing an entire bag of Raisinets or a quart of ice cream. No matter how bad it seems at the time, don't use it as an excuse to go off the program. Pretend you are a child leaning to walk. At first you fall a lot. What do you do? Pick yourself up. With time you will fall less. Ultimately, you won't fall at all.

In a way, the problem isn't the diet itself but rather your motivation to stay on the diet. It's really a psychological problem and should be treated this way. There are tricks to get yourself motivated. What is commonly called a set point should really be considered your habit point. The weight you are now is the result of a combination of habits based upon your heredity and your environment. Heredity—that tendency on your father's side for a pot belly or on your mother's side for a big behind—you can't change. The environment—your food and your exercise—you can change.

Your best motivator is self respect. You've got to care enough about yourself to do something about losing weight. Your motivator may be wanting to look better, which is a form of health—psychological health—or because your joints are hurting or because you have high blood pressure or diabetes.

Many commercial programs are available, such as Weight Watchers, Diet Center, Nutri/System, Optifast, and Jenny Craig. Costs range from a few hundred to a few thousand dollars for the programs, which provide psychological and nutritional counseling and, in some cases, food. TOPS (Take Off Pounds Sensibly) and Overeaters Anonymous are patterned after Alcoholics Anonymous. Long-term data are not available, but it is safe to say that most people who start a program drop out, do not achieve the results they want, or gain back the weight they lose within a year or two. They are not solutions you will stick with.

The Beverly Hills Diet, Immune Power Diet, Atkins Diet, and just about any other diet with a catchy name and a book on the best-seller list should be avoided. The only thing they have in common is their heavy advertising and long list of testimonials. The same warning should be heeded with dietary supplements.

Chromium picolinate, for example, is only the latest diet fad in a long history of diet fads. Because **chromium** helps metabolize sugar, this product is being touted for weight loss, cholesterol lowering, and control of diabetes. Combining **chromium** with picolinic acid to form chromium picolinate increases the absorption of the **chromium.**

Since it is sold as a food supplement rather than as as a drug, chromium picolinate is exempt from stringent FDA scrutiny. Still, this product cannot be recommended. Its value is unproven and it is potentially hazardous. **Chromium** is a trace element that is only important in the rare instances of chromium deficiency, which only occurs in severely malnourished infants. In these instances sugar metabolism is disturbed, but there is no evidence that chromium picolinate modifies sugar metabolism in otherwise healthy people.

Other nutritional gimmicks you might hear about or see advertised on radio or TV, such as starch blockers, fat absorbers, fat burners, and the like should also be viewed with extreme skepticism, particularly if the offer is good only while supplies last. Real doctors sometimes tout these products, but it should be remembered that they have a financial stake in the matter. Doctor recommended is a phrase that often doesn't mean a thing.

Exercise

Some people do find exercise to be the complete answer to their weight problem, but this is unusual. Sumo wrestlers and professional football linemen prove that you can be very active physically and still be as big as a tank. This is not to discourage anyone from exercise, because exercise is essential to one's health and is good for almost any disease. It helps you to look better and feel better. It is also an excellent adjunct to a weight-loss diet. It's just that for weight control, except in children and teenagers, it won't usually do the job by itself.

As with decreasing your food calories, increasing their expenditure through exercise is a habit. Those who keep at it longest—which is the goal—are those who enjoy it the most.

Step one is to find an exercise you like. There are many possibilities: hiking, gardening, jogging, skiing, swimming, climbing, tennis, squash, handball, dancing, aerobics, and weight lifting. Walking is excellent. You need only a comfortable pair of shoes (the well cushioned running shoes are the best), you can do it just about anywhere, and you can adjust your pace to take it easy or really knock yourself out. Walking is good also because it's easy on the the joints. It is also one of the weight bearing exercises; the others are jogging, aerobics, and weight training. These have been shown to decrease the risk of osteoporosis by increasing bone density.

Step two of the good exercise program is to start easy: you're in this for the long haul. If you've scheduled yourself for a twenty-minute walk and don't feel up to it, cut it in half and do ten minutes instead (or five, if that's all you can squeeze in; five minutes is better than no minutes). There are those who say that a little exercise does no good. This is ridiculous. *Any* exercise is good. At a certain point, when you begin to feel very tired or injured or depressed, lay off for a day, but never more than a day—you'll lose momentum.

Be honest with yourself before buying an exercise machine on the basis of a TV commercial, unless you need household junk for your next garage sale. Although they can provide excellent exercise, what you see on TV are smiling, happy people effortlessly stair-stepping, treadmilling, and ab-rolling their way to fitness. Now, *nobody* really smiles on a stair-stepper, treadmill, or ab-roller when they are working out, and you won't either. You want to find something that you can do over and over again, day in and day out, winter, spring, summer, and fall. Most modern gyms contain lots of different types of machines, rows of TV sets, and handsome bodies to keep you from becoming bored by it all. They also staff people with the expertise to recommend how to purchase the correct exercise machine and what features are desirable.

Table 15. Calories and exercise

Activity	Calories per 20 minutes
walking	100
tennis	130
cycling	140
swimming	160
cross county skiing	230
jogging	300

Recommendations

There is no quick and easy solution to being overweight.

When trying to cut down on food, don't keep high calorie items around the house.

Don't wait until you're hungry to eat. You're likely to be ravenous. Your body knows what you need and when: schedule your meals and snacks accordingly. Don't eat to satisfy your hunger but to eat what you planned to eat.

Glandular and hormonal troubles, like thyroid and adrenal disease, can cause obesity. If you suspect them as the culprit for your weight problems, consult your doctor. He or she can find out if you have them with a physical examination and a few tests.

Think in terms of the type of food intake and the kind and amount of exercise you can reasonably do for the rest of your life. You must modify your behavior, which is no easy thing. Start by nudging yourself in the right direction.

Don't be seduced by nonfat foods. Look at the label. Many nonfat items contain lots of calories. Cows and elephants subsist on a completely vegetarian low-fat diet.

If you are obese, you may be a candidate for prescription drug therapy.

Exercise more.

Eat less.

30

YEAST INFECTIONS

Although the term yeast infection is most often applied to conditions of the female genitals, such infections can occur elsewhere, including beneath the breasts and at the corners of the mouth. Uncircumscised men also may suffer from yeast infections under the foreskin of the penis.

These infections are almost always caused by *Candida* germs, which are normally present in certain areas of human skin and are kept in check by bacteria that are also found there. Bacteria and yeasts are natural enemies and keep each other in balance. Under certain conditions, the balance can be altered, and overgrowth of the *Candida* can occur.

What alters the balance? Antibiotics, diabetes, pregnancy, and injury in the form of sexual intercourse are the most common causes. Individuals undergoing chemotherapy and those with AIDS are also susceptible. Some individuals just seem to be prone to develop these problems.

The most common symptoms of vaginal yeast infections are:

- Burning, itching, and redness of the skin of the vulva
- A thick, white, cheesy discharge which is typically *odorless*. If the discharge smells, it is more likely a bacterial infection, which can't be treated without a doctor's prescription.

Most women experience a vaginal yeast infection at least once in their lifetime, but fewer suffer recurrent infections.

If you have been diagnosed previously with a yeast infection, have responded to treatment, and the symptoms are identical to those you had before, you can safely treat yourself again. Several prescription anti-yeast drugs are also available, the most convenient being a single oral dose of fluconazole (Diflucan).

There are currently four OTC vaginal yeast infection products, **clotrimazole** (Gyne-Lotrimin and Mycelex-7), **miconazole** (Monistat 7), **butoconazole** (Femstat 3), and **tioconazole** (Vagistat-1). Medically, they are more or less interchangeable, and generics are available, so buy whatever is on sale that day. Although different forms are available, such as creams, tablets, and prefilled applicators, the best bet is probably one of the combination products, such as the Mycelex-7 Combination-Pack. This product includes seven tablets and seven grams of cream to treat the vagina itself and the skin simultaneously for a full week. The one- or three-day regimens, such as the **tioconazole** and **butoconazole** programs, might be more convenient. Whatever you choose, make sure that the product contains at least one of the above active ingredients. Some, such as Yeast-Gard, do not.

If redness and itching of the vulva itself are pronounced, you can alleviate the symptoms somewhat by applying a small amount of one-percent **hydrocortisone** cream twice a day *in addition* to the anti-yeast medication. *Do not* apply the **hydrocortisone** by itself or you'll make the yeast infection worse.

Some studies show that eating eight ounces of yogurt a day helps prevent vaginal yeast infections, as well as vaginal bacterial infections (make sure the yogurt has active *Lactobacillus acidophilus).* If you decide on this and are watching your weight, use the nonfat variety with an artifical sweetener, because the calories and fat can add up.

Don't attempt to prevent yeast, bacterial, or other infections by douching. The vagina, like other organs of the body, tends to take care of itself and to be self-cleaning. The natural secretions contain substances that help keep tissue moist and healthy.

Commercial douches contain a vast array of ingredients like **povidone-iodine, octoxynol-9, cetylpyridinium chloride, sodium bicarbonate, methyl salicylate, phenol, thymol, men-**

thol, boric acid, benzoic acid, benzethonium chloride, and vinegar, along with a host of other chemicals. There really is no valid reason to use any of them, and douching with anything is not recommended. If you have a yeast infection you should treat it appropriately; if you're using a douche for birth control, it is a terrible method; if you're trying to prevent sexually transmitted diseases you're fooling yourself; if you have vaginal odor, see a doctor.

INGREDIENTS

○ ○ ○

Acetaminophen

ooo

Use
Internal analgesic (reduces pain) and antipyretic (reduces fever). There is no effect on inflammation.

Where found
Although the brand name Tylenol is practically synonymous with this drug, acetaminophen is found in many other products, such as Acetaminophen Uniserts (suppositories), Actamin products, Alka-Seltzer (some), Aminofen, Anacin Aspirin Free, Aspirin Free Arthritis Pain Formula, Aspirin Free Pain Relief, Bromo-Seltzer, Dynafed EX, Dyspel, Excedrin products (sometimes with **aspirin**), Feverall, Liquiprin, Midol, Percogesic, Stanback AF Extra-Strength, Tapanol, Tempra, Valorin, XS Hangover Relief, and generics. In addition, it is present in many combination cough and cold concoctions, along with antihistamines, decongestants, cough suppressants, and expectorants.

Recommended dosage
Adults and children over 12 years: 325 to 650 mg every 4 hours. Do not take more than 4 gm (4000 mg) per day.

Children 11 to under 12 years: 480 mg every 4 to 6 hours. Do not take more than 5 doses a day.

Children 9 to under 11 years: 400 mg every 4 to 6 hours. Do not take more than 5 doses a day.

Children 6 to under 9 years: 320 mg every 4 to 6 hours. Do not take more than 5 doses a day.

Children 4 to under 6 years: 240 mg every 4 to 6 hours. Do not take more than 5 doses a day.

Children 2 to under 4 years: 160 mg every 4 to 6 hours. Do not take more than 5 doses a day.

The dosage for children under 2 should be determined by your doctor. Check with your doctor before taking acetaminophen if you are pregnant or nursing. Do not take for longer than 10 days for pain or 3 days for fever.

Side effects and overdosage

Generally well tolerated. Liver damage is a rare but serious complication that has been reported in those who consume large amounts of alcohol or who take larger than recommended amounts. It is important to seek medical attention immediately in case of a suspected overdose, because the toxic effects can be partially reversed if treated early enough. Furthermore, symptoms of overdose may be delayed for two to three days. Early signs of liver damage include nausea, vomiting, sweating, and weakness. Later signs include yellowness (jaundice) of the whites of the eyes or skin. Allergic reactions, such as rash, itching, or hives are rare, as are kidney damage and interference with blood clotting. Drug interactions may occur with the anticoagulant (blood thinner) warfarin and with certain drugs used to treat tuberculosis.

Activated charcoal

ooo

Use

Adsorbent for use in poisoning. It is sometimes recommended for vague abdominal complaints and excess gas, but there is little objective evidence that it alleviates such symptoms. It is also used as a deodorizer in some ostomy products.

Where found

Actidose, Charcoaid G, Insta-Char, Liqui-Char. In combination with sorbitol in Actidose with Sorbitol and Insta-Char With Sorbitol. Liqui-Char is available with and without sorbitol. Activated charcoal is not simple charcoal; you cannot manufacture it yourself by burning toast.

Recommended dosage

Follow manufacturer's recommendations. Activated charcoal is available either as a powder you mix yourself or as a prepared suspension. In general, the maximum amount is 10 gm per day in divided doses, not to exceed 7 days. Do not attempt to administer it to anyone who is unconscious.

Side effects and overdosage
Generally safe, but since activated charcoal is not selective, it can bind and inactivate other medications. May also cause vomiting or constipation and color the stool black. Aspiration into the lungs can be fatal.

Alcohol

ooo

Use
Antiseptic and delivery vehicle for drugs. Strictly speaking, the term alcohol refers to ethanol, or grain alcohol. When purchased for external use it is often denatured with chemicals that make it unfit for consumption. Unfortunately, these chemicals also irritate the skin. Isopropyl alcohol—commonly referred to as rubbing alcohol—is similar, although a different chemical. Cetearyl alcohol and cetyl alcohol are sometimes found in products designed for external use.

Where found
Numerous cough and cold liquids, first-aid products, ear drops, mouthwashes, oral discomfort liquids, and external skin products.

Recommended dosage
Follow manufacturer's recommendations.

Side effects and overdosage
High concentrations of alcohol, especially if applied repeatedly, may dry and irritate the skin. Mouthwashes containing alcohol are suspected of contributing to oral cancer. The alcohol in cough and cold remedies can be mildly intoxicating. Alcohol is highly flammable.

Synonyms
Ethanol.

Alginic acid

OOO

Use
A compound derived from algae that is used along with an antacid to form a jelly-like substance with the stomach contents. This jelly is then supposed to float on top of the stomach contents like a raft. Alginic acid is also sometimes used to thicken or stabilize skin creams.

Where found
Gaviscon product line and generics.

Recommended dosage
Follow manufacturer's recommendations.

Side effects and overdosage
Safe when used as directed.

Synonyms
Magnesium alginate, sodium alginate.

Allantoin

OOO

Use
Skin softener and protectant. The substance is widely distributed in plants and animals.

Where found
Many creams and ointments used as moisturizers and protectants.

Recommended dosage
Follow manufacturer's recommendations. By itself may be applied as often as needed in a 0.5 to 2 percent strength.

Side effects and overdosage
Very safe.

Aloe

OOO

Use
Stimulant laxative. Also used as a natural external remedy for various skin ailments, although there is no reliable evidence that it works.

Where found
Nature's Remedy, with **cascara sagrada**.

Recommended dosage
Follow manufacturer's recommendations. Do not use in pregnancy.

Side effects and overdosage
Aloe as a laxative is much too irritating to the intestine to be recommended.

Synonym
Aloe vera.

Alpha-galactosidase

OOO

Use
Anti gas. Works by breaking down complex sugars so they cannot be fermented by intestinal bacteria.

Where found
Beano liquid or tablets.

Recommended dosage
Adults and children over 12 years: 3 to 8 drops of liquid added to the first bite of gas-forming food. Add after food has cooled so as not to inactivate the enzyme. For tablets, take 2 to 3 with the first mouthful. You can chew them,

crush them, or swallow them whole. One tablet of Beano equals 5 drops.

Side effects and overdosage
Well tolerated in recommended doses. May increase blood sugar if you have diabetes. Avoid if you are allergic to molds or have galactosemia. (There is one isolated report of someone who developed an intestinal perforation after several weeks of taking Beano, but the two events may not have been related.)

Aluminum acetate

○○○

Use
Astringent, usually in solution form. Best for skin rashes that are oozing, weeping, or blistered, such as poison ivy or chickenpox. Sometimes used in ear drops to provide an acidic environment hostile to germs. Also sometimes incorporated into creams or lotions.

Where found
Domeboro and Bluboro are composed of **aluminum sulfate** and **calcium acetate,** which, when mixed with water, produce aluminum acetate.

Recommended dosage
For Domeboro: mix one or two effervescent tablets or packets in water. The resulting solution can be used as a soak or compress. For a compress, soak an old handkerchief or similar soft cotton cloth in the solution, wring it out, and apply for 15 to 30 minutes, 3 or 4 times a day. Do not use on excessively dry skin. Do not use for longer than 7 days.

Side effects and overdosage
Excessive use can dry out and irritate the skin.

Synonym

Burrow's solution. Aluminum subacetate (basic aluminum acetate) is similar but is formed by the reaction of aluminum sulfate and acetic acid.

Aluminum carbonate

OOO

Use
Antacid, relatively low strength.

Where found
Basaljel.

Recommended dosage
Variable. If taking on your own, follow the directions on the label, and if you experience relief, stop. If taking on the advice of a doctor for ulcers or other symptoms, follow instructions.

Side effects and overdosage
See **aluminum hydroxide.**

Aluminum chloride

OOO

Use
Antiperspirant. Stronger and generally more effective than cosmetic antiperspirant products.

Where found
Certain Dri (12.5 percent solution in water).

Recommended dosage
Apply sparingly once a day at bedtime. Once perspiration is under control decrease frequency of applications. Discontinue if irritation develops.

Side effects and overdosage
May sting and cause skin irritation.

Aluminum chlorohydrate

○○○

Use
Antiperspirant and astringent. Similar to **aluminum chloride** but less irritating.

Where found
Many antiperspirants in a variety of forms.

Recommended dosage
Follow manufacturer's recommendations.

Side effects and overdosage
Well tolerated.

Synonyms
Aluminum chlorohydrex, aluminum dichlorohydrate, aluminum dichlorohydrex, and aluminum sesquichlorohydrex. The terms PEG (**polyethylene glycol**) and PG (**propylene glycol**) are sometimes found following these chemical names.

Aluminum hydroxide

○○○

Use
Antacid, relatively low strength.

Where found
See antacid chart in Chapter 16. May be combined with **simethicone**. Also found in certain buffered **aspirin** products, such as Maximum Strength Ascriptin and Cama Arthritis Pain Reliever.

Recommended dosage

Highly individual. Follow manufacturer's directions. For adults with heartburn the usual dose is 2 teaspoons (of suspension) or 1 to 2 tablets 5 to 6 times a day or at bedtime as needed. Do not take for longer than 2 weeks. In general it is best to space administration of other medications with antacids for 2 hours. In the case of ciprofloxacin (Cipro) and other quinolone antibiotics, antacids should be taken at least 6 hours before or 2 hours after the antibiotic. Many drug interactions are possible. Most of the time, aluminum hydroxide decreases the absorption of the drug, but it increases the absorption of valproic acid (Depakene) and diazepam (Valium).

Side effects and overdosage

Constipation. For this reason, aluminum salts are often coupled with magnesium salts. Use with caution if you have recently experienced severe intestinal bleeding or if you have decreased kidney function. May also lead to low phosphate or the milk-alkali syndrome.

Aluminum oxide

ooo

Use

Dentifrice abrasive.

Where found

Colgate Baking Soda & Peroxide Whitening Toothpaste.

Recommended Dosage

Follow manufacturer's recommendations.

Side effects and overdosage

Generally well tolerated.

Aluminum silicate

○○○

Use
Dentifrice abrasive.

Where found
Caffree Anti-Stain Toothpaste and Dentu-Creme.

Recommended Dosage
Follow manufacturer's recommendations.

Side effects and overdosage
Generally well tolerated.

Aluminum sulfate

○○○

Use
Ingredient mixed with **calcium acetate** and water to form **aluminum acetate,** an astringent. Also used as an antiperspirant buffered with sodium aluminum lactate.

Where found
Bluboro, Domeboro, Pedi-Boro. With **hydrocortisone** in Bactine Hydrocortisone and Cortizone cream products. With **phenol** and **camphor** in Ostiderm.

Recommended dosage
Follow manufacturer's recommendations.

Side effects and overdosage
Generally well tolerated, but if the compound is used by itself it can be very irritating to the skin.

Ammonia water

000

Use
Counterirritant in external analgesics. More potent than household ammonia but is mixed with oleic acid and sesame oil to form a type of soap or liniment. Aromatic ammonia spirit (smelling salts) is a related substance.

Where found
After-Bite.

Recommended dosage
Apply to affected areas 3 to 4 times a day as needed.

Side effects and overdosage
Should be applied carefully only to the involved areas. Inhalation of vapors can be highly irritating to the mucous membranes, causing eye irritation, sneezing, and coughing. In the available concentrations it is well tolerated, but in high concentrations ammonia can cause severe breathing difficulties and eye problems, including temporary blindness.

Synonyms
Stronger ammonia water, stronger ammonium hydroxide solution, spirit of hartshorn.

Ammonium chloride

000

Use
Diuretic (promotes excretion of water), usually used for menstrual cramps. In the body the chloride ion combines with the sodium to form sodium chloride (salt), which is excreted along with water. This process, however, cannot maintain itself, and unlike other diuretics, ammonium

chloride stops working after several days. It can also be used to make the urine more acidic.

Where found
Generic tablets.

Recommended dosage
1 gm 3 times a day. Do not use for longer than 6 days.

Side effects and overdosage
Do not use if you have liver or kidney disease. May cause nausea and upset stomach. In higher than recommended amounts acid may accumulate, causing the condition called acidosis.

Antazoline

ooo

Use
Antihistamine in eye care products.

Where found
Vasocon-A (with naphazoline).

Recommended dosage
Follow manufacturer's recommendations. Do not use if you have narrow angle glaucoma. Discontinue and see your doctor if you experience eye pain, changes in vision, continued redness or irritation of the eye, or if your condition worsens or persists for longer than 72 hours.

Side effects and overdosage
May sting or burn when applied.

Aspirin

ooo

Use
Internal analgesic. Reduces pain, fever, and inflammation (redness, tenderness, swelling, and stiffness). Also used as a blood thinner (anticoagulant) to prevent heart attacks, strokes, and TIAs (transient ischemic attacks).

Where found
The Bayer company discovered aspirin and still produces vast amounts of it. It is also present in Anacin, Anodynos, Alka-Seltzer (some), Ascriptin, Aspercin, Aspergum, Aspermin, Aspirtab, Back-Quell, BC products, Buffaprin, Buffasal, Bufferin, Buffinol, Cope, Ecotrin, Emagrin, Excedrin, Goody's products, Halfprin, Heartline, Norwich Aspirin, St. Joseph, Stanback, Supac, and Vanquish, alone or in combination with other ingredients, such as acetaminophen, caffeine, salicylamide, and antihistamines. Some preparations include buffering antacids, such as aluminum hydroxide, sodium bicarbonate, calcium carbonate, or magnesium salts. Others are enteric coated, which delays the digestion of the product so that it is broken down in the small intestine rather than in the stomach. Rectal suppositories are available.

Recommended dosage
Adults and teenagers over 15 years: 650 to 1000 mg every 4 to 6 hours. Do not take more than 4000 mg (4 gm) a day. Take with food, antacid, or a full glass of water to reduce stomach upset. For use as a blood thinner 81 mg a day (one baby's aspirin) is enough. Do not give to children or teenagers 15 years of age or younger. Be very careful with alcohol intake. If you consume more than 3 drinks a day, you probably shouldn't be taking *any* oral OTC pain reliever. Also, do not take aspirin with other pain relievers. Be particularly careful if you are taking blood thinners (anticoagulants) such as warfarin (Coumadin), since the combination can cause serious bleeding. Also be careful with high blood pressure medications (such as ACE inhibi-

tors), heart medications, water pills (diuretics), methotrexate, probenecid, and anticonvulsants. **Methylcellulose** laxatives, such as Citrucel, can decrease aspirin absorption. Although the analgesic effect of aspirin is relatively fast, the antiinflammatory effect works slowly. Taking the maximum OTC dose, it generally takes 3 to 4 days for aspirin—measured by salicylate levels in the blood—to achieve an antiinflammatory effect. The regular dose of an aspirin tablet is 325 mg. The extra strength type is 500 mg, and there is a low dose of 81 mg. The maximum allowable OTC dose in all cases, however, remains the same, at 4000 mg. A timed release form is available that can be taken every 8 hours as opposed to every 4 hours. Avoid during pregnancy, particularly during the last 3 months. Do not take for longer than 10 days for pain or 3 days for fever.

Side effects and overdosage
The most common side effect is upset stomach, including pain, heartburn, nausea, diarrhea, and gas. A more serious side effect is the production of new stomach ulcers or the reactivation of old stomach ulcers. Intestinal bleeding can occur without your knowing that it is happening, even with buffered or enteric coated products. By far the most serious side effect—Reye's syndrome—is in children and teenagers who have been given aspirin to treat flu symptoms or chickenpox. Reye's syndrome causes liver and brain damage and is potentially fatal. Its early symptoms are vomiting and neurological signs, such as listlessness, disorientation, or aggressive behavior.

High doses of aspirin may produce dizziness or ringing in the ears, particularly if you ingest other sources of salicylates, such as raisins, prunes, licorice, tea, or **bismuth subsalicylate** (Pepto-Bismol). Another potential source of salicylates is from skin absorption by applying **methyl salicylate** found in many external pain relievers such as BenGay and Mentholatum. Potentially serious allergies to aspirin, including hives and wheezing, can occur, especially in those with asthma or nasal polyps. Do not take aspirin if you have gout or high uric acid in your blood.

Synonyms
Acetylsalicylic acid, ASA.

Attapulgite

○○○

Use
Anti-diarrheal that works by adsorption. Over thirty times more adsorbent than kaolin. It is usually referred to as activated attapulgite, which means that it has been heated; this increases its ability to adsorb. Attapulgite itself is a type of clay used in fertilizers, pesticides, and drugs. It is also the major ingredient in kitty litter.

Where found
Diasorb, Donnagel, Kaopectate products, Parepectolin, Rheaban, and generics.

Recommended dosage
Recommended doses vary slightly depending upon whether you take the liquid suspension, tablets, or chewable tablets. The general range is as follows: Adults and children 12 years of age and older: 1200 to 1500 mg after each loose bowel movement, not to exceed 9000 mg per day. Children 6 to 12: 600 mg after each loose bowel movement, not to exceed 4200 mg per day. Children 3 to 6: 300 mg after each loose bowel movement, not to exceed 2100 mg per day. Doses for children less than 3 should be determined by a doctor. Do not take for longer than 2 days unless your doctor directs otherwise.

Side effects
Safe when used as directed, but may cause constipation, bloating, and abdominal fullness.

Synonyms
Activated attapulgite, purified hydrated magnesium aluminum silicate.

Avobenzone

○○○

Use
Sunscreen, mainly for the UVA band of ultraviolet light.

Where found
Shade UVAGuard.

Recommended dosage
Sunscreens should be applied generously covering every square inch of exposed skin surface at least one half hour before sun exposure. Anywhere from 1 to 2 ounces is usually needed for the entire body.

Side effects and overdosage
May cause irritation and sun sensitivity.

Bacitracin

○○○

Use
Antibiotic effective against certain (gram positive) bacteria.

Where found
Baciguent and generics. With **polymyxin B** in Betadine First Aid Antibiotics and Polysporin. With **polymyxin B** and **neomycin** in various triple antibiotics such as Betadine First Aid, Campho-phenique Triple Antibiotic, Clomycin, Lana-biotic, Mycitracin, Neosporin, Tri-Biozene, and Tribiotic Plus.

Recommended dosage
Apply 1 to 3 times a day. May be applied directly to a cut, abrasion, or other wound and to the surrounding skin.

Side effects
May cause local skin irritation.

Bentoquatam

○○○

Use
Barrier for toxic plants (poison ivy, poison oak, and poison sumac).

Where found
IvyBlock (with alcohol).

Recommended dosage
Shake bottle and apply to skin 15 minutes prior to expected exposure, leaving a smooth wet film. Not for children under the age of 6 years unless directed by your doctor. Avoid contact with eyes. May be reapplied in 4 hours or as needed to maintain protection. Do not use if you already have poison ivy.

Side effects and overdosage
May dry and irritate skin. Solution is flammable before it dries.

Synonym
Quaternium-18 bentonite.

Benzalkonium chloride

○○○

Use
Antiseptic and preservative. It also lowers surface tension (detergent). It is in the general class of quaternary ammonium compounds, along with benzethonium chloride and methylbenzethonium chloride.

Where found
Numerous compounds possess varying concentrations. A .01 to 0.1 percent solution can be used to cleanse skin and wounds. A .02 to .05 percent solution is present in some

vaginal douches. Very dilute solutions can be used to irrigate the bladder. It is also present in creams for diaper dermatitis, shampoos, herpes medications, spermicides, and eye drops.

Recommended dosage
Follow instructions for the parent compound.

Side effects and overdosage
Benzalkonium chloride can be irritating in concentrated solutions if used over a long period. It is poisonous if large amounts are taken internally.

Benzethonium chloride
OOO

Use
Antiseptic and preservative.

Where found
Clinical Care Wound Cleanser, Formula Magic Antibacterial Powder, Orchid Fresh II Perineal/Ostomy Cleanser, and many other skin, eye, and vaginal douche products.

Recommended dosage
Follow manufacturer's directions.

Side effects and overdosage
Generally safe but may cause irritatation.

Benzocaine
OOO

Use
Local anesthetic of the ester type.

Where found

Widely used in many sore throat lozenges, canker sore and toothache medications, hemorrhoid preparations, burn ointments, and poison ivy products, such as Aerocaine, Americaine, Anbesol, Baby Gumz, Benzodent Denture Analgesic, Bicozene, Bi-Zets, Boil Ease, Burntame, Cepacol (some), Cetacaine, Chloraseptic, Dentapaine, Dent's Toothache products, Dermoplast, Foille products, Hurricaine, Isodettes, Kank-A, Lagol, Lanacane, Lipmagik, Medadyne, Medicated First Aid Burn Cream, Medicone, Numz-it, Orabase (most), Orajel (most), Palmer's Skin Success, Protac, Red Cross Canker Sore Medication, Rhuli, Solarcaine, Spec-T, Sting-Eze, and Zilactin. Also found in some vaginal creams and in creams designed to prolong erections, as in Maintain.

Recommended dosage

Follow manufacturer's recommendations.

Side effects and overdosage

May cause irritation and allergic contact dermatitis.

Synonym

Ethyl aminobenzoate.

Benzoic acid

○○○

Use

Antiseptic. It is found with **salicylic acid** in Whitfield's ointment, an old antifungal preparation.

Where found

Femizol-M, Rid-Itch, Summer's Eve (some), and mouthwashes.

Recommended dosage

Follow manufacturer's recommendations.

Side effects and overdosage
Generally safe.

Benzoin
ooo

Use
Protectant for skin and mucous membranes. It is a sticky brown resin, derived from pine trees, that dries to form a protective coating.

Where found
Generic products.

Recommended dosage
For mucous membranes such as the mouth. Adults and children over 6: apply every 2 hours, as needed. Dry the area before application.

Side effects and overdosage
May cause allergic skin irritation (contact dermatitis).

Synonyms
Tincture of benzoin (solution in alcohol), compound tincture of benzoin (mixture of benzoin, storax, balsam, and aloe in alcohol).

Benzoyl peroxide
ooo

Use
Anti acne topical medication. Promotes peeling (keratolytic) and has antiseptic qualities.

Where found
Ambi 10 Acne Medication, Benoxyl, Clearasil (some), Ex-ACT (some), Fostex BPO, Loroxide, Neutrogena Acne

Mask, On-The-Spot, Oxy (some), Palmer's Skin Success Invisible Acne Medication, PanOxyl, Persa-Gel, Vanoxide, and generics. Available in creams and cleansers, usually in a 5 to 10 percent concentration.

Recommended dosage
Apply 1 to 2 times a day to the entire affected area. Do not spot treat individual lesions.

Side effects and overdosage
The most common side effect is skin irritation: redness, burning, itching, and scaling. This may occur in almost anyone if enough benzoyl peroxide is applied. In laboratory experiments on mice it has promoted tumor growth, but there is no evidence that it does the same in humans. Still, the compound is undergoing continued FDA scrutiny and has been placed in Category III—insufficient data for a final determination of safety and effectiveness.

Benzyl alcohol
ooo

Use
Local anesthetic used for mucous membranes. Found naturally in jasmine, hyacinth, and other plants. It acts quickly but only lasts about 10 to 30 minutes. Much less effective than other local anesthetics, such as **benzocaine** or **lidocaine**. Also used as a preservative in foods, drugs, and cosmetics.

Where found
Hemorrhoid products: Anusol Suppositories, Hydrosal Hemorrhoidal, Tucks Clear Gel. Also in some mouthwashes, sprays, and lozenges in .05 to 10 percent strengths.

Recommended dosage
Follow manufacturer's recommendations.

Side effects and overdosage
Safe in recommended strengths.

Biotin

OOO

Use
A B vitamin that is essential to general metabolism. Deficiency is rare but symptoms of it may be nausea, vomiting, weakness, aches and pains, loss of appetite, anemia, depression, skin rashes, a sore tongue, and heart problems. It can be caused by malnutrition or by eating large quantities of *raw* egg whites without the yolks. The egg white contains a protein that binds to the biotin and prevents it from being absorbed.

Where found
Liver, kidneys, egg yolk, dark green vegetables, cauliflower, salmon, carrots, bananas, soy flour, and yeast. It is also manufactured by bacteria in the intestine. Present in many multivitamin products.

Recommended dosage
Recommended daily allowances (mg) for adults and children over 4: 0.3; children under 4: 0.15; infants: .05.

Side effects
There are no reports of toxicity from high doses.

Bisacodyl

OOO

Use
Stimulant type laxative. Usually works in 6 to 10 hours orally and 15 to 60 minutes rectally.

Where found
Bisco-Lax, Correctol, Dulcolax, Evac-Q-Kwik suppositories, Feen-A-Mint, Fleet products (many), Gentle Laxative, and generics. May be found in some products combined with other laxatives or with the stool softener **docusate**.

Recommended dosage

Oral: adults and children over 12 years: 10 to 30 mg.; children 6 to under 12 years: 5 to 10 mg. Rectal: adults and children over 2: 10 mg.; children under 2: 5 mg. Bisacodyl tablets are enteric coated to avoid stomach irritation and stomach upset. Do not chew or crush them. Also do not take them with antacids or histamine receptor antagonists (**ranitidine, famotidine, cimetidine,** or **nizatidine**). Do not use for more than 1 week.

Side effects and overdosage

Well tolerated in recommended doses. If used in high doses or for long periods of time it may cause severe diarrhea with loss of fluids, electrolytes (body salts), calcium, and protein. Suppositories may cause a burning sensation in the rectum.

Bismuth subgallate

OOO

Use

Deodorizer for those with colostomies.

Where found

Devko (with **activated charcoal**), Devrom Chewable Tablets.

Recommended dosage

Follow manufacturer's recommendations.

Side effects and overdosage

Well tolerated in recommended doses.

Bismuth subsalicylate

OOO

Use

Upset stomach (heartburn, indigestion, and nausea) and diarrhea (particularly infectious diarrhea). Also often used in combination with antibiotics and stomach acid suppressants such as proton pump inhibitors or histamine receptor antagonists in the eradication of the *Helicobacter pylori* bacterium, which causes most stomach ulcers

Where found
Pepto-Bismol products and generics.

Recommended dosage
Liquid: adults and children over 12 years: 2 tablespoons every ½ to 1 hour as needed, not to exceed 16 tablespoons of regular strength or 8 tablespoons of the concentrated liquid per day; children 9 to under 12 years: ½ the adult dose; children 6 to under 9 years: 2 teaspoons every ½ to 1 hour as needed, not to exceed 16 teaspoons of the regular strength or 8 teaspoons of the concentrated liquid per day; children 3 to under 6 years: 1 teaspoon every ½ to 1 hour as needed, not to exceed 8 teaspoons of the regular strength or 4 teaspoons of the concentrated liquid per day; children under 3 years: dose is based on body weight. Follow manufacturer's recommendations. Tablets: adults and children over 12 years: 2 tablets every ½ to 1 hour as needed, not to exceed 16 tablets per day; children 9 to under 12 years: 1 tablet every ½ to 1 hour, not to exceed 8 tablets per day. Follow your doctor's recommendations if being used to treat stomach ulcers. The dose is generally 2 tablets 4 times a day for 1 to 2 weeks, depending upon the other medications being used. Do not use this or other salicylates in pregnancy, particularly in the last 3 months. They also pass into breast milk and should be avoided if you are nursing.

Side effects and overdosage
Small doses are well tolerated, but as with other salicylates, side effects increase with higher doses, especially in the young or the elderly. People allergic to **aspirin** and NSAIDs (**ibuprofen, ketoprofen,** and **naproxen**) may cross react with this product. Never give a salicylate to children or teenagers under the age of 16 years with fever, symptoms of the flu, or chickenpox because of the possibly causing Reye's syndrome. May cause constipation in children and older adults, which may be severe. Drug interactions may occur with anticoagulants, oral antidiabetic drugs, **aspirin,**

NSAIDS, probenecid (Benemid), sulfinpyrazone (Anturane), and tetracyclines. Bismuth subsalicylate may aggravate gout and may increase bleeding in those with hemophilia or other bleeding problems. Those with kidney disease should be careful because of decreased excretion. May aggravate stomach ulcers and may interfere with urine sugar tests, especially if taken in large amounts. Overdosage may cause seizures, hearing loss, confusion, ringing or buzzing in the ears, severe drowsiness, tiredness, excitement, nervousness, and fast or deep breathing. Some people may notice a temporary darkening of the tongue or green, gray, or black stool.

Boric acid

OOO

Use
Preservative and buffer (adjusts acidity). Although used as an antiseptic in vaginal douches and eye preparations, it is not effective for these purposes.

Where found
Vaginal douches, eye drops, eye ointments, contact lens products, ear drops.

Recommended dosage
Follow manufacturer's recommendations.

Side effects and overdosage
Well tolerated in amounts present in most manufactured products but may be toxic if large amounts are absorbed.

Brompheniramine

OOO

Use
Antihistamine (H_1 receptor) in the alkylamine class.

Where found

Most of the Dimetane and Dimetapp product lines contain this antihistamine. Some others that contain it alone or in combination are Bromfed, Dristan Cold Multi-Symptom Maximum Strength, and Vicks DayQuil 12-Hour Allergy Relief.

Recommended dosage

Adults and children over 12 years: 4 mg every 4 to 6 hours as needed. Do not take more than 24 mg per day. Children 6 to under 12 years: ½ the adult dose. Children 2 under 6 years: ¼ the adult dose. Take with food if stomach upset is a problem. Avoid if you are pregnant.

Side effects and overdosage

Generally well tolerated and less sedating than **diphenhydramine**. Some side effects, such as drowsiness, are undesirable when you are taking it during the day and want to stay awake, but desirable when you are taking it to go to sleep. Similarly, a dry nose may be uncomfortable unless you have a cold. Uncommon side effects include allergies, itching, rash, abnormal sensitivity to sunlight (photosensitivity), sweating, chills, nervousness, excitability (especially in children), blurred vision, upset stomach, nausea, vomiting, constipation, diarrhea, difficulty with urination, thickening of lung secretions, and wheezing. Older people are more sensitive to these side effects. The sedative effect can be marked with alcohol, so avoid this combination. Don't take any antihistamine if you have glaucoma, heart disease, thyroid disease, an enlarged prostate, diabetes, or high blood pressure. For lung diseases such as asthma, emphysema, or chronic bronchitis, ask your doctor. Also do not take antihistamines with other sleeping aids, tranquilizers, or antidepressants such as monoamine oxidase inhibitors (MAOIs).

Butamben

OOO

Use
Local anesthetic for minor burns. Does not penetrate un-damaged skin well and so is not useful unless there has been an injury.

Where found
Butesin Picrate ointment.

Recommended dosage
Apply 3 to 4 times a day as needed. Do not use for longer than 7 days.

Side effects and overdosage
Generally safe in recommended doses but may cause skin irritation. Turns skin and bandages yellow.

Synonym
Butamben picrate.

Butoconazole

OOO

Use
Vaginal antifungal and antiyeast (Candida) in the azole class.

Where found
Femstat 3.

Recommended dosage
Femstat 3 comes with a disposable applicator and detailed instructions for use. Do not use with tampons or in girls under the age of 12 years. Do not use if you are pregnant or if you have abdominal pain, fever, or a foul smelling discharge.

Side effects and overdosage
Generally well tolerated.

Synonym
Butoconazole nitrate.

Caffeine

ooo

Use
General nervous stimulant. It also opens the breathing passages, increases breathing rate and heart rate, reduces blood flow to the liver and brain, and promotes urination.

Where found
As the sole active ingredient: 20/20, 357 Magnum II, Caffedrine, Dexitac, Enerjets, High Gear, King of Hearts, NoDoz, Overtime, Pep-Back, Quick Pep, Vivarin, and generics. Also found in many combination pain relievers (internal analgesics) and cough, cold, and allergy products. It is included in some menstrual products for its diuretic action.

Recommended dosage
Adults over 18 years: 100 to 200 mg every 3 to 4 hours, as needed. Avoid if you are pregnant or nursing.

Side effects and overdosage
Side effects of caffeine are highly variable and depend upon how much is ingested and how sensitive you are to its effects. High doses can cause nervousness, insomnia, tremor, dizziness, ringing in the ears, nausea, diarrhea, vomiting, heart palpitations, rapid heart rate, excessive urination, and upset stomach. The upset stomach is increased if caffeine is taken with **aspirin, ibuprofen, ketoprofen, naproxen,** or **alcohol.** The metabolism of caffeine is inhibited by **cimetidine,** some antibiotics, estrogen, and **alcohol.** Caffeine decreases the absorption of iron from food. Excessive caffeine taken during pregnancy has been linked to low

birth weight infants. Caffeine is secreted in a mother's milk, so that infants nursing from mothers who take in too much caffeine may become irritable and restless.

Calcium acetate

○○○

Use
Mixed with **aluminum sulfate** and water to form **aluminum acetate,** an astringent.

Where found
Bluboro and Domeboro. With **hydrocortisone** in Cortizone creams.

Recommended dosage
Follow manufacturer's recommendations.

Side effects and overdosage
Well tolerated.

Calcium carbonate

○○○

Use
Antacid, toothpaste abrasive, and calcium supplement (insoluble). Moisture absorber in powders. Often derived from oyster shells and contains 40 percent calcium.

Where found
Many antacids (see Chapter 16), toothpastes, skin protectant powders, and nutritional supplements.

Recommended dosage
For antacid use, follow manufacturer's recommendations. In general, it is best to allow 1 or 2 hours to elapse between taking antacids and taking other medications. In the case of

ciprofloxacin (Cipro) and other quinolone antibiotics, antacids should be taken at least 6 hours before or 2 hours after the antibiotic. When used as a calcium supplement it is best taken with food.

Recommended daily allowances (gm): adults and children over 4: 1.2; children under 4: 0.8; infants: 0.6; pregnant and nursing women: 1.3.

Side effects and overdosage
Usually well tolerated but excessive amounts (over 2 gm a day) can increase blood calcium and cause constipation, urinary problems, headache, loss of appetite, mood changes, muscle pain, twitching, nausea, vomiting, nervousness, and fatigue. Large doses may also lead to kidney stones and kidney damage. Avoid inhaling the powdered form.

Calcium citrate

OOO

Use
Calcium supplement (soluble). Contains 21 percent calcium.

Where found
Citracal. Chewy Bears and Citron contain it as well as calcium carbonate.

Recommended dosage
See calcium carbonate for calcium requirements. May be taken on an empty stomach.

Side effects and overdosage
See calcium carbonate.

Calcium gluconate

OOO

Use
Calcium supplement (soluble). Contains 9 percent calcium.

Where found
Neo-Calglucon syrup. Calcet, Calci-Caps, and a few other vitamin and mineral products contain this form of calcium as well as other forms.

Recommended dosage
See **calcium carbonate** for calcium requirements. May be taken on an empty stomach.

Side effects and overdosage
See calcium carbonate.

Calcium lactate

OOO

Use
Calcium supplement (soluble). Contains 21 percent calcium.

Where found
This calcium salt is found in a few combination vitamin and mineral products.

Recommended dosage
See **calcium carbonate** for calcium requirements. May be taken on an empty stomach.

Side effects and overdosage
See calcium carbonate.

Calcium phosphate

OOO

Use
Calcium supplement (insoluble) derived from bone meal.
Contains 39 percent calcium.

Where found
Posture and a few other combination nutritional supplements.

Recommended dosage
See **calcium carbonate** for calcium requirements. Take with
meals.

Side effects and overdosage
See calcium carbonate.

Synonym
Dicalcium phosphate.

Calcium polycarbophil

OOO

Use
Bulk forming laxative and diarrhea control drug. Highly
absorbent, able to soak up 60 times its weight in water. As a
laxative it usually works in 12 to 24 hours but may take as
long as three days. The calcium portion allows the polycarbophil to be manufactured as a liquid.

Where found
As a laxative in FiberCon, Konsyl Fiber, and Mitrolan. For
diarrhea control in Equalactin.

Recommended dosage
For the laxative effect the dose should be individualized.
The adult dose is 1 to 6 gm a day as needed, but follow

manufacturer's directions for the recommended dose and for use in children. Always take with at least 8 oz of water, fruit juice, soda, or other liquid. More liquid is even better. Do not use for longer than 1 week. Do not take if you have difficulty swallowing. The usual dose for diarrhea in adults is 4 to 6 gm a day, usually by tablet.

Side effects and overdosage
The most serious side effect is blockage of the esophagus or choking if not enough fluid is taken. This ingredient also contains calcium, some of which is absorbed into the bloodstream (see **calcium carbonate**).

Synonym
Polycarbophil.

Camphor

ooo

Use
In low (0.1 to 3 percent concentrations) it is used as an external analgesic, anesthetic, and anti-itch ingredient. In higher concentrations (3 to 11 percent) it functions as a counterirritant analgesic, something that irritates and confuses the nerve endings. Also available as a topical cough suppressant and in combination with **phenol** as an antiseptic. It is derived from the camphor tree and is also produced synthetically.

Where found
Camphor is widely used in the OTC drug industry, although it is not as prevalent as **menthol**, with which it is often combined. Many combination external analgesics, cough and cold remedies, and sore throat products contain it, such as Banalg, Betuline, Blue Star, Deep-Down, Flexall Ultra Plus, Minit-Rub, Noxzema Original, Pain-X, Sarna, Soltice, and TheraPatch. It is also present as a local anesthetic in Pazo ointment (with **ephedrine** and **zinc oxide**), a hemorrhoidal preparation.

Recommended dosage
Follow manufacturer's recommendations.

Side effects and overdosage
Camphor in recommended doses is relatively safe, but there are reports of toxicity, especially with large doses, in children. Breathing problems and seizures can occur from applying high concentrations over wide areas. The American Academy of Pediatrics recommends that products containing camphor not be used at all in children. Further, one of the FDA's committees has recommended that concentrations no higher than 2.5 percent be available OTC. At the present time, however, this limit is not observed. Because there are more effective ingredients, it is probably best to stay away from products with concentrations of camphor higher than 2.5 percent, such as ArthriCare Double Ice Pain Relieving Rub, Ultra Strength Bengay Nongreasy Pain Relieving cream, Campho-phenique Pain Relieving Antiseptic, Dencorub, Heet, Mentholatum, Numol, Vicks Vapo-Rub, and Vicks VapoSteam.

Capsaicin

ooo

Use
Pain relief, particularly that due to shingles, diabetes, and arthritis. It is derived from chili peppers.

Where found
Arthur Itis, Capzasin products, Dencorub, Dolorac, Double Cap, Flexcin, Icy Hot Arthritis Therapy Gel, Zostrix products, and generics. Combination products with other counterirritants are available, such as in Absorbine Arthritis Strength, ArthriCare Pain Relieving Rub, ArthriCare Ultra, Heet, Menthacin, Pain-X, and Sloan's Liniment.

Recommended dosage
Rub well into the affected area until it disappears. Wash your hands thoroughly—unless you're using it for hand

pain. In that case, don't wash it off for at least 30 minutes, but in the meanwhile be very careful not to touch the mucous membranes of your eyes, nose, mouth, or genitals. Do not use with a heating pad or hot compress. The area may be left uncovered or a loose fitting bandage may be applied. Do not use in children under 2 years or on broken or irritated skin. Continue to apply it 2 to 4 times a day until you experience relief. With arthritis, you should get some relief in 2 weeks but for the neuralgia of shingles and diabetes it may take 2 to 4 weeks. With neuralgias of the head and neck it may take even longer, up to 4 to 6 weeks. Once it does relieve pain, you have to continue to use it regularly 3 or 4 times a day to prevent a recurrence, although if you stop and your pain returns, you can begin using it again.

Side effects and overdosage
Expect a warm, stinging, or hot sensation at first. This is normal, although if the sensation is severe or accompanied by redness, you should stop. After a while, the warm sensation should disappear, at which time the drug will begin to work. Trying to decrease this side effect by applying less cream or fewer applications may delay its effectiveness.

Synonyms
Capsicum, capsicum oleoresin.

Carbamide peroxide

OOO

Use
Ear wax softening agent in ear drops and wound cleanser in canker sore products. It is similar to **hydrogen peroxide** in that it effervesces and releases oxygen when brought into contact with tissue. The **urea** portion of the compound helps to soften skin and wound debris.

Where found
In ear preparations: Auro, Aurocaine, Debrox, Dent's Ear Wax Drops, E.R.O., and Murine Ear Wax Removal System. In canker sore preparations: Cankaid, Gly-Oxide, and Orajel Perioseptic.

Recommended dosage
For ear wax removal: adults over 12 years: 5 drops in affected ear(s) 2 times a day as needed. Leave in place for 15 minutes. Do not use for longer than 4 days. Some products come with a soft rubber irrigating syringe. For canker sore treatment: adults and children over 2 years: apply 2 to 3 drops to affected areas 4 times a day as needed. Do not use for longer than 7 days.

Side effects and overdosage
Generally well tolerated when used as recommended. Will cause stinging and pain when applied to canker sores.

Synonym
Urea hydrogen peroxide.

Carnitine

OOO

Use
A nutritional compound essential for general metabolism. Deficiency of it is extremely rare but may occur in very ill infants on prolonged intravenous feeding. Symptoms may include weakness, liver and heart problems, and impaired carbohydrate metabolism.

Where found
Meats (especially red) and nutritional supplements. The main source is through synthesis in the body from amino acids.

Recommended dosage

There is no recommended daily allowance. Supplements are available in several dosage strengths.

Side effects and overdosage

No reports of toxic effects have been reported from doses as high as 15 gm per day.

Casanthranol

ooo

Use

Stimulant type laxative, usually effective in 8 to 12 hours.

Where found

In combination with the stool softener **docusate** in Docusate Potassium with Casanthranol, Laxative & Stool Softner, Peri-Colace, and Regulace.

Recommended dosage

Follow manufacturer's directions for the combination products. Usual adult dose is 30 to 60 mg as needed. Do not use for longer than 1 week. Avoid if you are pregnant or nursing.

Side effects and overdosage

May cause nausea, abdominal pain or cramping, diarrhea, or rash.

Cascara sagrada

ooo

Use

Stimulant type laxative that usually is effective in 6 to 8 hours. This is an old remedy obtained from buckthorn tree bark, which American Indians used to call sacred bark. It is in the anthraquinone laxative category along with **senna**.

Where found
By itself in many generic products called cascara sagrada or cascara sagrada aromatic fluidextract. Also in combination with **magnesium hydroxide** in milk of magnesia cascara and with **aloe** in Nature's Remedy.

Recommended dosage
Adults and children over 12 years: 2 to 6 milliliters of aromatic fluidextract; 300 mg to 1000 mg of the solid form. Children 2 to under 12 years: ½ of adult dose. Liquid forms are more reliable and preferable. Do not use for longer than 1 week. Avoid in pregnancy.

Side effects and overdosage
Prolonged use may cause pigmentation of the colon and discolor the urine.

Castor oil
ooo

Use
Stimulant type laxative, usually effective in 2 to 6 hours. Unlike other stimulant laxatives castor oil acts in the small intestine (as opposed to the large intestine) and is converted to a different chemical, ricinoleic acid, which is the actual laxative.

Where found
Emulsoil, Kellogg's Tasteless Castor Oil, Neoloid, Purge, and generics.

Recommended dosage
Follow manufacturer's recommendations, since some products do not contain 100 percent castor oil. For pure castor oil, the usual doses are: adults and children over 12 years: 15 to 60 milliliters (1 to 4 tablespoons); children 2 to under 12 years: 5 to 15 milliliters (1 to 3 teaspoons); children under 2 years: 1 to 5 milliliters ⅕ to 1 teaspoon). Do not use for longer than 1 week. It is most effective on an empty

stomach. The unpleasant taste may be improved by chilling and adding to a glass of fruit juice or soda. Do not take at bedtime because it usually acts quickly and you'll have to get up in the middle of the night. Avoid if you are pregnant.

Side effects and overdosage
May cause cramping. Prolonged use may result in dehydration and electrolyte (body salt) imbalance.

Cellulose ethers

OOO

Use
Demulcent (mucous membrane protectant) in artificial tears and artificial salivas.

Where found
Artificial tears: Celluvisc, Comfort Tears, GenTeal Lubricant, Isopto Tears, Ocurest, Refresh Plus, Tearisol, Ultra Tears. Also found in other artificial tear products combined with dextran, **povidone**, and **glycerin**. Artificial salivas: Glandosane Mouth Moisturizer, Moi-Stir, Optimoist, Oralbalance, Salivart Synthetic Saliva.

Recommended dosage
Eyes: 1 or 2 drops in affected eyes as needed. Mouth: follow manufacturer's recommendations.

Side effects and overdosage
None reported.

Synonyms
Hydroxypropyl methylcellulose, hydroxyethylcellulose, hydroxypropyl cellulose, methylcellulose, and carboxymethylcellulose.

Cetylpyridinium chloride

OOO

Use
Antiseptic quat (quaternary ammonium compound) with detergent action (lowers surface tension).

Where found
In the following vaginal douches, oral care products, and first aid creams: Cepacol products, First Aid Cream, some Massengill products, Mycinettes, Protac, Oral-B Anti-Plaque Rinse, Plus White Anti Stain Oral Rinse, Cool Peppermint Scope, Swish, Tech 2000, Spectro-Jel.

Recommended dosage
Follow manufacturer's recommendations.

Side effects and overdosage
May cause skin and mucous membrane stinging, burning, and irritation; may stain teeth and increase tartar formation.

Chlorhexidine

OOO

Use
Antiseptic and preservative.

Where found
Betasept Surgical Scrub, Hibiclens, Hibistat. Some contact lens disinfectants. Also in the prescription oral care product Peridex.

Recommended dosage
Follow manufacturer's recommendations.

Side effects and overdosage
Generally well tolerated but can damage the eyes. In oral products it tastes bitter and can stain the teeth, in addition to increasing the buildup of tartar (calculus).

Synonym
Chlorhexidine gluconate.

Chlorobutanol

○ ○ ○

Use
Antiseptic and preservative.

Where found
A few nasal sprays and contact lens solutions contain this preservative.

Recommended dosage
Follow manufacturer's recommendations.

Side effects and overdosage
Generally well tolerated.

Chlorothymol

○ ○ ○

Use
Antiseptic effective against bacteria and fungi that is related to **phenol**.

Where found
Lanacane Creme (with **benzethonium chloride** and **benzocaine**) and Rid-Itch Liquid (with **benzoic acid** and **resorcinol**).

Recommended dosage
Follow manufacturer's recommendations.

Side effects and overdosage
May cause skin irritation.

Chloroxylenol

○○○

Use
Antibacterial and antifungal. Currently in the FDA Category III (insufficient data on safety and effectiveness).

Where found
Barri-Care Antimicrobial Barrier, Care Creme Antimicrobial, Foille products (some), Lobana Peri-Gard, Medicated First Aid Burn Cream, Vaseline Medicated Antibacterial Petroleum Jelly, Zeasorb powder.

Recommended dosage
Follow manufacturer's recommendations.

Side effects and overdosage
Generally well tolerated when used as directed.

Chlorpheniramine

○○○

Use
Antihistamine (H_1 receptor) in the alkylamine class.

Where found
Chlor-Trimeton is virtually synonymous with this very popular antihistamine. Some other products that contain it are A.R.M., many Alka-Seltzer allergy products, Allerest (most), BC Allergy Sinus Cold, Cerose-DM, Cheracol Plus, Codimal, Comtrex (most), Contac (some), Coricidin,

Creomulsion, Dallergy-D, Demazin, Dristan Cold Multi-Symptom, Duadacin, Efidac 24 Chlorpheniramine, Fedahist, Flu-Relief, Genamin, Gencold, Gendecon, Hayfebrol, Histatab Plus, Kolephrin, Kophane, Napril, Novahistine, PediaCare (some), Protac SF, Scot-Tussin DM, Sinapils, Sinarest (most), Sine-Off Sinus Medicine, Singlet, Sinulin, Sinutab Maximum Strength Sinus Allergy, Teldrin, Tetrahist, TheraFlu (most), Tri-Nefrin, Triaminic (some), Triaminicin, Triaminicol, Tricodene (most), Tylenol products (many), and Vicks product line (many). Often the combinations include **pseudoephedrine, guaifenesin, dextromethorphan,** and **acetaminophen.**

Recommended dosage

Adults and children over 12 years: 4 mg every 4 to 6 hours. Do not take more than 24 mg in 24 hours. Children 6 to under 12 years: ½ the adult dose. Children 2 to under 6 years: ¼ the adult dose. Timed release products are available to give 8 mg for 8 hour relief and 12 mg for 12 hour relief. Food intake does not matter, but you can take it with food if it upsets your stomach. Avoid if you are pregnant or nursing.

Side effects and overdosage

Generally well tolerated and less sedating than **diphenhydramine.** Some side effects, such as drowsiness, are undesirable when you are taking it during the day and want to stay awake, but desirable when you are taking it to go to sleep. Similarly, a dry nose may be uncomfortable unless you have a cold. Uncommon side effects include allergies, itching, rash, abnormal sensitivity to sunlight (photosensitivity), sweating, chills, nervousness, excitability (especially in children), blurred vision, upset stomach, nausea, vomiting, constipation, diarrhea, difficulty with urination, thickening of lung secretions, and wheezing. The sedative effect can be marked with alcohol, so avoid this combination. Older people are more sensitive to these side effects. Don't take any antihistamine if you have glaucoma, heart disease, thyroid disease, an enlarged prostate, diabetes, or high blood pressure. Also do not take antihistamines with other sleeping aids, tranquilizers, or antidepressants such as monoamine oxidase inhibitors (MAOIs). For use in lung diseases such as asthma, emphysema, or chronic bronchitis, check with your doctor.

Choline salicylate

ooo

Use
Relieves pain, inflammation, and fever. Similar to **aspirin** but less effective.

Where found
Arthropan Liquid.

Recommended dosage
Adults and children over 15 years: 435 to 870 mg every 4 hours as needed, not to exceed 5325 mg a day. Do not give to children or teenagers 15 years of age or younger with symptoms of the flu or chickenpox. Do not take for longer than 3 days for fever or 10 days for pain. Take with food or water but not with antacids (will increase the fishy odor of the product). Avoid if you are pregnant or nursing.

Side effects and overdosage
In general these are similar to **aspirin,** except that there is much less of a tendency to blood thinning.

Chromium

ooo

Use
Chromium is a chemical element that is present in very small amounts in the body but is important in sugar (glucose) and insulin metabolism. Although inadequate chromium causes sugar imbalance, chromium deficiency is very uncommon except in the unusual circumstance where an extremely malnourished infant has been fed with insufficient chromium in the diet.

Where found
Liver, fish, grains, milk. Chromium picolinate is available in 200 mcg tablets.

Recommended dosage
Estimated recommended daily allowances (mcg): adults and children over 12 years: 50 to 200; Children 1 to 6: 20 to 120; Infants: 10 to 60.

Side effects and overdosage
Excessive amounts can cause breathing difficulties and lung cancer. Extremely high levels may produce kidney disease, liver disease, and convulsions. Chromium toxicity is usually seen in those who have had industrial exposure to it. There are two forms in which chromium can enter the body, the trivalent and the hexavalent. The former is relatively safe whereas the latter can cause toxicity. Chromium supplementation is currently all the rage, but perhaps by the time you read this the fad will have abated. See Chapter 29 on weight reduction for more information.

Cimetidine
ooo

Use
Reduces stomach acid by blocking the histamine$_2$ receptor. Used for the prevention and relief of heartburn, indigestion, and sour stomach.

Where found
Tagamet HB 200.

Recommended dosage
Adults and children over 12 years: take 200 mg 2 times a day. Do not take more than 400 mg a day. May be taken with or without food. Do not take for longer than 2 weeks and do not take if you are nursing. Check with your doctor if you have liver or kidney disease.

Side effects and overdosage
In OTC approved doses, cimetidine is well tolerated. In higher prescription doses, such as 400 mg four times a day, side effects may include diarrhea, dizziness, skin rash,

swollen breasts, nausea, vomiting, headache, confusion, drowsiness, hallucinations, and sexual dysfunction. Many drug interactions are possible. Antacids decrease the absorption of cimetidine, as do certain prescription drugs. Cimetidine *increases* the effects of **alcohol, caffeine,** oral antidiabetes drugs, certain tranquilizers and antidepressants, calcium channel blockers, narcotics, the blood thinner warfarin, and tetracycline, among many others. It *decreases* the effects of the heart medication digoxin.

Citric acid

○○○

Use

A compound derived from citrus fruits such as oranges, tangerines, lemons, and grapefruit that has several uses. For antacid use it is often combined with **sodium bicarbonate.** When water is added the concoction fizzes and the result of the chemical reaction is that the citric acid is converted to **sodium citrate** and the **sodium bicarbonate** is converted to sodium carbonate and carbon dioxide. Medically, citric acid solutions are sometimes used to dissolve kidney stones, to reduce the acidity of the urine, and to treat metabolic acidosis. It is also an alpha hydroxy acid that may be used to soften the skin.

Where found

Alka-Seltzer and similar generic products. External preparations include: Acid Mantle Creme, Aveeno Gentle Skin Cleanser Lotion, and Oilatum soap. Also found in several eye products as a buffer to adjust acidity.

Recommended dosage

Follow manufacturer's recommendations.

Side effects and overdosage

When used orally with **sodium bicarbonate** it should be used with care in those on salt restriction because of the sodium content. In skin care products it is generally well tolerated. If citric acid by itself is ingested in large doses it can erode tooth enamel and be locally irritating.

Clemastine

ooo

Use
Antihistamine (H_1 receptor) in the ethanolamine class. It is long acting.

Where found
Contac 12 Hour Allergy, Tavist-1, and Tavist-D (with **phenylpropanolamine**).

Recommended dosage
Adults and children over 12 years: 1 mg every 12 hours as needed, not to exceed 2 mg a day. Food intake does not matter, but take with food if it upsets your stomach. Avoid if you are pregnant or nursing.

Side effects and overdosage
Generally well tolerated, but of the antihistamines, clemastine in particular has been shown to harm nursing infants. Some side effects, such as drowsiness, are undesirable when you are taking it during the day and want to stay awake, but desirable when you are taking it to go to sleep. Similarly, a dry nose may be uncomfortable unless you have a cold. Uncommon side effects include allergies, itching, rash, abnormal sensitivity to sunlight (photosensitivity), sweating, chills, nervousness, excitability (especially in children), blurred vision, upset stomach, nausea, vomiting, constipation, diarrhea, difficulty with urination, thickening of lung secretions, and wheezing. The sedative effect can be marked with **alcohol,** so avoid this combination. Older people are more sensitive to these side effects. Don't take any antihistamine if you have glaucoma, heart disease, thyroid disease, an enlarged prostate, diabetes, or high blood pressure. Also do not take antihistamines with other sleeping aids, tran-

quilizers, or antidepressants such as monoamine oxidase inhibitors (MAOIs). Check with your doctor before using an antihistamine if you have a lung disease such as asthma, emphysema, or chronic bronchitis. Clemastine may worsen symptoms in those with porphyria.

Clotrimazole

OOO

Use
Topical antifungal used to treat ringworm, jock itch, athlete's foot, sun fungus (tinea versicolor), and vaginal yeast infections. It is a member of the imidazole (azole) class of antifungals.

Where found
Cruex (some), Desenex (some), Femizol-7, Gyne-Lotrimin, Lotrimin (some), Mycelex (some), Mycelex-7, generics.

Recommended dosage
For creams, lotions, and solutions, apply a small amount and rub in twice a day. Keep away from your eyes. For vaginal yeasts, follow the package instructions.

Side effects and overdosage
Allergies are uncommon. Discontinue if you experience increased redness, blisters, or a burning sensation.

Coal tar

OOO

Use
Dandruff, seborrhea, and psoriasis control. Crude coal tar consists of about 10,000 different chemicals and is obtained by distilling and refining coal.

Where found

Balnetar, Cutar, Denorex products, DHS Tar, Doak Oil, Doak Tar, Doctar, Duplex-T, Estar, Glover's products (most), Grandpa's Pine Tar products, Ionil-T, MG217 for Psoriasis, Neutrogena T/Gel, Oxipor VHC, Pentrax, Polytar, Psoriasin, Psoriasis Tar, psoriGel, Sebutone, SLT Lotion, Taraphilic, Tarsum, Tegrin, Vanseb-T, X-Seb T, Zetar.

Recommended dosage

Follow manufacturer's recommendations. These will vary depending upon whether you are using a liquid, bath oil, gel, soap, or shampoo. Avoid in areas where skin meets skin, such as the groin or armpits. In hairy areas apply in the general direction of hair growth (with the grain rather than against it) to avoid getting the material into hair follicles.

Side effects and overdosage

May cause significant irritation and actual aggravation of the skin condition. Folliculitis (inflammation of the hair follicles), increased sensitivity to sunlight (photosensitivity), and discoloration of the skin and hair are also possible. It is also possible to absorb some of the active chemicals in coal tar after skin applications; some of these compounds are potentially carcinogenic.

Cocoa butter

ooo

Use

A solid fat that is a major constituent of chocolate. It is derived from the roasted seeds of *Theobroma cacao* (cacao). Often employed as a basis for suppositories and hemorrhoidal preparations and as a skin protectant in diaper rash products. In pure form it has a reputation for improving scars and abnormal skin pigmentation, but there is no evidence that it helps these conditions.

Where found
Cocoa butter is combined with other protectants in several hemorrhoidal products, such as Preparation H suppositories. It is also a minor ingredient in Diaper Guard. Many generic preparations are available.

Recommended dosage
In pure form may be applied as often as needed. When combined with other ingredients, follow manufacturer's recommendations.

Side effects and overdosage
Very safe.

Synonym
Theobroma oil.

Cod-liver oil

○○○

Use
Skin protectant derived from the fresh livers of cod and other fish. Also used as a source of **vitamins** A and D.

Where found
A and D Medicated Ointment, Care-Creme, Desitin, and many other skin care products. Available in generic form as a nutritional supplement.

Recommended dosage
Follow manufacturer's recommendations.

Side effects and overdosage
Safe for external use. Some may find the odor objectionable.

Codeine

O O O

Use
Cough suppressant. It is a relative of opium with similar but weaker activity than morphine. It is also available in higher prescription doses for pain management, often combined with **acetaminophen** (Tylenol with codeine).

Where found
Only available in some states OTC, and in those states certain additional controls are required.

Recommended dosage
Adults and children over 12 years: 10 to 20 mg every 4 hours, not to exceed 120 mg a day. Children 6 to under 12 years: ½ the adult dose.

Side effects and overdosage
Constipation is relatively common in recommended doses. Allergic skin rashes are possible. Codeine may cause drug dependence in some individuals, although the tendency for this is not great.

Synonyms
Codeine phosphate, codeine sulfate.

Copper

O O O

Use
Present in the body in trace amounts, copper is critical to many biochemical reactions. Its functions are complex and intertwined with the metabolism of **zinc.** Ingestion of excess **zinc,** for example, can cause copper deficiency. Deficiency, although rare, may also be seen in infants on prolonged

intravenous feedings or during times of famine. The most important feature of copper deficiency is decreased absorption of iron.

Where found
Liver, shellfish, grains, beans, peas, nuts, and nutritional supplements.

Recommended dosage
Recommended daily allowances (mg): adults and children over 4: 2; children under 4: 1; infants: .6.

Side effects and overdosage
Copper toxicity may cause nausea, vomiting, diarrhea, anemia, convulsions, and intestinal hemorrhage.

Cornstarch

○○○

Use
Dusting powder and protectant. Sometimes mixed with **zinc oxide** or other substances. Highly absorbent.

Where found
Present in many commercial preparations for external use.

Recommended dosage
Apply to skin as often as needed but avoid breathing in particles.

Side effects and overdosage
Although it was once thought that cornstarch supports the growth of germs, recent evidence indicates that this is not the case.

Synonym
Topical starch.

Cromolyn

○○○

Use
Hay fever (allergic rhinitis) control. Works by stabilizing mast cells and preventing the release of histamine, but is not an antihistamine. It is also available by prescription in inhalers, eye drops, and pills.

Where found
Nasalcrom nasal solution.

Recommended dosage
Adults and children over 6 years: 1 spray in each nostril every 3 to 4 hours, not to exceed 6 doses a day. Blow your nose first. Best taken regularly starting a week before and during the allergy season.

Side effects and overdosage
The most common side effects are stinging, burning, or irritation of the nose. Sneezing sometimes occurs immediately after instillation. Nosebleeds, postnasal drip, and skin rashes have occurred, as have severe allergic reactions, but it is generally well tolerated.

Synonym
Cromolyn sodium, sodium cromoglycate.

Cyclizine

○○○

Use
Antihistamine for control of nausea and vomiting and motion sickness. A member of the piperazine class of antihistamines, like meclizine, but shorter acting.

Where found
Marezine.

Recommended dosage

Adults and children over 12 years: 50 mg every 4 to 6 hours as needed, not to exceed 200 mg a day. Children 6 to under 12 years: 25 mg every 6 to 8 hours as needed, not to exceed 75 mg a day. Not recommended for children under 6. Avoid during pregnancy.

Side effects and overdosage

Generally well tolerated with less sedation than some other histamines. Besides drowsiness, dryness of the nose and mouth is relatively common. Uncommon side effects include allergies, itching, rash, abnormal sensitivity to sunlight (photosensitivity), sweating, chills, nervousness, excitability (especially in children), blurred vision, upset stomach, nausea, vomiting, constipation, diarrhea, difficulty with urination, thickening of lung secretions, and wheezing. The sedative effect can be marked with alcohol, so avoid this combination. Older people are more sensitive to these side effects. Don't take any antihistamine if you have glaucoma, thyroid disease, an enlarged prostate, diabetes, or high blood pressure. Also do not take antihistamines with other sleeping aids, tranquilizers, or antidepressants such as monoamine oxidase inhibitors (MAOIs). For lung diseases such as asthma, emphysema, or chronic bronchitis, check with your doctor. Cyclizine may aggravate heart failure and heart attacks. It has also been used illicitly; tablets have sometimes been used to make injectable substances.

DEET

ooo

Use

Insect repellent effective against a wide variety of insects.

Where found

Ben's, Bug Stuff, Cutter, Muskol, Off!, Repel, and Skedaddle! products. Highest concentration (100 percent) is found in Repel 100. Also present in a number of suncreens, such as Coppertone Bug & Sun, Snoopy Sunblock SPF 15 Plus

Insect Protection, Solar Gel SPF 15 Plus Insect Protection, and Sun & Bug Stuff.

Recommended dosage

Apply to clothing prior to exposure. Although it may also be applied to skin, avoid the areas around the eyes and where skin meets skin, as in the groin or armpits, because of irritation.

Side effects and overdosage

May irritate skin. Although generally safe, there have been occasional cases of damage to the nervous system, heart, and blood vessels. This has occurred with ingestion, inhalation of vapors, and absorption through contact with the eyes and skin. Children in particular may develop serious reactions. Seizures, coma, shock, and death have been reported.

Synonym

Diethyltoluamide, N,N-diethyl-meta-toluamide.

Desoxyephedrine

OOO

Use

Decongestant that works by narrowing blood vessels as a vasoconstrictor. This compound is related to the amphetamines.

Where found

Vicks Vapor Inhaler.

Recommended dosage

Adults and children over 12 years: 2 inhalations every 2 hours as needed. Children 6 to under 12 years: ½ the adult dose under adult supervision.

Side effects and overdosage

May cause burning, stinging, sneezing, increased nasal discharge, and irritation. Do not use if you have heart disease, high blood pressure, thyroid disease, diabetes, or an enlarged prostate. Rebound congestion, in which reflex dilatation of blood vessels causes persistant nasal stuffiness despite ever increasing doses, may occur.

Synonym
Levodesoxyephedrine.

Dexbrompheniramine

OOO

Use
Antihistamine (H_1 receptor) in the alkylamine class.

Where found
Most products in the Drixoral line contain this antihistamine in combination with various combinations of **pseudoephedrine, acetaminophen,** and **dextromethorphan.** 12-Hour Cold Tablets and Disophrol Chronotabs Sustained Action Cold & Flu combine it with **pseudoephedrine.**

Recommended dosage
Adults and children over 12 years: 2 mg every 4 to 6 hours, not to exceed 12 mg a day. Children 6 to under 12 years: ½ the adult dose. Children 2 to under 6 years: ¼ the adult dose. Food intake does not matter, but take with food if it upsets your stomach. Avoid if you are pregnant or nursing.

Side effects and overdosage
Generally well tolerated and less sedating than **diphenhydramine.** Some side effects, such as drowsiness, are undesirable when you are taking it during the day and want to stay awake, but desirable when you are taking it to go to sleep. Similarly, a dry nose may be uncomfortable unless you have a cold. Uncommon side effects include allergies, itching, rash, abnormal sensitivity to sunlight (photosensitivity), sweating, chills, nervousness, excitability (especially in children), blurred vision, upset stomach, nausea, vomiting, constipation, diarrhea, difficulty with urination, thickening

of lung secretions, and wheezing. The sedative effect can be marked with **alcohol,** so avoid this combination. Older people are more sensitive to these side effects. Don't take any antihistamine if you have glaucoma, heart disease, thyroid disease, an enlarged prostate, diabetes, or high blood pressure. For lung diseases such as asthma, emphysema, or chronic bronchitis, check with your doctor. Also do not take antihistamines with other sleeping aids, tranquilizers, or antidepressants such as monoamine oxidase inhibitors (MAOIs).

Synonym
Dexbrompheniramine maleate.

Dextromethorphan

○ ○ ○

Use
Cough suppressant related to codeine and morphine but with much less tendency toward drug dependence.

Where found
By itself in products such as Benylin Adult Cough Formula, Buckley's Mixture, Cough-X, Creo-Terpin, Diabe-tuss DM, Hold, Pertussin, Pinex, Robitussin (some), Scot-Tussin (some), Spec-T Sore Throat Cough Suppressant, Tetra Formula, Soothing Vicks 44 Cough Relief, and in combination with decongestants, antihistamines, internal analgesics, and mucus liquefiers (expectorants) in numerous cough, cold, and allergy products.

Recommended dosage
Adults and children over 12 years: 10 to 20 mg every 4 to 8 hours, not to exceed 120 mg per day. Children 6 to under 12 years: ½ the adult dose. Children 2 to under 6 years: ¼ the adult dose. Avoid if you are pregnant or nursing. Check with your doctor if you have asthma or liver disease. Do not take for longer than 7 days unless your doctor directs otherwise.

Side effects and overdosage
Well tolerated in recommended doses but may cause drowsiness or stomach upset. If taken for a long time may cause habituation. Do not take with the antidepressants known as monoamine oxidase inhibitors (MAOIs) such as Nardil (phenelzine), or for two weeks after stopping an MAOI: deaths have been reported from this drug interaction.

Synonyms
Dextromethorphan hydrobromide, dextromethorphan polistirex.

DHEA
ooo

Use
"Fountain of Youth." The benefits claimed for DHEA include strengthened immune system, increased sex drive, and improved circulation, among many others. Studies in rats show a possible anti-obesity effect, but there is no evidence of this in humans.

Where found
Multiple sources. It should be noted that Mexican or wild yams *(Dioscorea mexicana* and *villosa)* do *not* contain DHEA.

Recommended dosage
Unknown.

Side effects and overdosage
Large doses can cause virilization—production of male characteristics such as increased facial hair and deepening of the voice—in women. There has been at least one reported case of hepatitis and there is evidence that some women might be at risk for increased rates of ovarian cancer. Nothing is known about the long-term effects.

Synonyms
Dehydroepiandosterone, dehydroepiandosterone sulfate, prasterone, dehydroandosterone.

Dibucaine

○○○

Use
Local anesthetic of the amide type. Sometimes used to produce spinal anesthesia.

Where found
Hemorrhoidal: Nupercainal ointment.

Recommended dosage
Adults and children over 12 years: Apply a 0.25 to 1 percent concentration 3 to 4 times a day as needed.

Side effects and overdosage
May cause contact dermatitis (irritation of the skin).

Dicalcium phosphate

○○○

Use
Abrasive in toothpastes and calcium supplement.

Where found
Various toothpastes, vitamin, and calcium products.

Recommended dosage
Follow manufacturer's recommendations.

Side effects and overdosage
Usually well tolerated but excess ingested calcium can cause constipation, difficult or painful urination, frequent urge to urinate, headache, loss of appetite, mood or mental

changes, muscle pain or twitching, nausea, vomiting, nervousness, slow breathing, unpleasant taste, and fatigue.

Dimenhydrinate
ooo

Use
Antihistamine of the ethanolamine class used to prevent motion sickness and nausea. It is thought to act by depressing the motion center in the middle ear. It is the **diphenhydramine** salt of 8-chlorotheophylline.

Where found
The name Dramamine is most often associated with this drug, but it is also found in Calm X and Triptone.

Recommended dosage
Adults and children over 12 years: 50 to 100 mg every 4 to 6 hours, not to exceed 400 mg per day. Children 6 to under 12 years: 25 to 50 mg every 6 to 8 hours, not to exceed 150 mg per day. Children 2 to under 6 years: 12.5 to 25 mg every 6 to 8 hours, not to exceed 75 mg per day. Tablets, chewable tablets, and liquids are available. Take with food if it upsets your stomach. Avoid if you are pregnant or nursing.

Side effects and overdosage
See **diphenhydramine**.

Synonym
Diphenhydramine theoclate.

Diphenhydramine
ooo

Use
Antihistamine in the ethanolamine class. It is the most widely used and versatile antihistamine and is used to

control allergies, coughs, and nausea. It is also employed as a sleeping aid and, externally, as a local anesthetic.

Where found

The brand name Benadryl is virtually synonymous with diphenhydramine, both in internal and external forms, but it is also found in dozens of products. It can be purchased in pure form—the best way—or in various cough and cold remedies, sleeping aids, and antiemetics for control of motion sickness. Some other internal products that contain it, alone or in combination, are: Aller-med, Anacin P.M. Aspirin Free, Arthriten PM, Backaid PM, Bayer products (some), Compoz, Diphenadryl, Doan's P.M. Extra Strength, Dormarex, Dormin, Excedrin PM, Genahist, Hydramine, Legatrin PM, Midol PM Night Time Formula, Nauzene, Nervine Nighttime Sleep-Aid, Nytol, Scott-Tussin (some), Sleep Rite, Sleepinal, Snooze Fast, Sominex, Tranquil, Twilite, Tylenol product line (some), Unisom Pain Relief, Unisom Sleepgels. A variety of capsules, tablets, caplets, and liquids are available. Externally, some products that contain it are: Cala-gel, Dermamycin, Dermapax, Dermarest, Di-Delamine, HC-Dermapax, Hydrosal, and Ivarest 8-Hour Medicated Cream.

Recommended dosage

As an oral antihistamine: adults and children over 12 years: 25 to 50 mg every 4 to 6 hours, not to exceed 300 mg per day; children 6 to under 12 years: ½ the adult dose; children 2 under 6 years: 6.25 mg every 4 to 6 hours, not to exceed 37.5 mg per day. As a sleep aid: adults and children over 12 years: 50 mg taken 30 minutes before bedtime. To prevent motion sickness: adults and children over 12 years: 25 mg taken 30 minutes before departure. In all cases, food intake does not matter. Take with food if it upsets your stomach. Externally: follow manufacturer's recommendations. Avoid if you are pregnant or nursing.

Side effects and overdosage

Whether a given effect of diphenhydramine is a side effect depends upon your reason for taking it. As a general rule, diphenhydramine and other antihistamines are well tolerated. Some effects, such as drowsiness, are undesirable when you are taking it during the day and want to stay awake, but desirable when you are taking it to go to sleep. Similarly, a dry nose may be uncomfortable unless you have a cold. Many other side effects have been reported, however, including itching, rash, abnormal sensitivity to sunlight (photosensitivity), sweating, chills, nervousness, excitability (especially in children), blurred vision, upset stomach, nausea, vomiting, constipation, diarrhea, difficulty with urination, thickening of lung secretions, and wheezing. The sedative effect can be marked with **alcohol,** so avoid this combination. Older people are more sensitive to these side effects. Don't take any antihistamine if you have glaucoma, heart disease, thyroid disease, an enlarged prostate, diabetes, or high blood pressure. If you have a lung disease such as asthma, emphysema, or chronic bronchitis check with your doctor. Also do not take antihistamines with other sleeping aids, tranquilizers, or antidepressants such as monoamine oxidase inhibitors (MAOIs). The most common side effect of diphenhydramine applied to the skin is an allergic irritation. Allergies to the drug in this form, in fact, are much more common than allergies to it in oral form.

Synonyms
Diphenhydramine hydrochloride. For **diphenhydramine citrate** see below.

Diphenhydramine citrate

○○○

Use
Antihistamine.

Where found
Excedrin PM and Goody's PM (both with **acetaminophen**).

Recommended dosage

Adults and children over 12 years: 38 to 76 mg every 4 to 6 hours. Do not take more than 456 mg a day. Children 6 under 12 years: ½ the adult dose. Children 2 to under 6 years: ¼ the adult dose. Avoid if you are pregnant or nursing.

Side effects and overdosage

See **diphenhydramine**.

Docusate

000

Use

Stool softener that is a wetting agent (detergent), helping water and fat in feces to mix and thus to pass more easily. Usually works in 1 to 3 days but may take as long as 5 days. Docusate sodium has been used also to soften ear wax, but is not approved for that purpose.

Where found

By itself: Colace, Correctol Stool Softener, Dialose, Ex-Lax Stool Softener, Regulax SS, Sof-lax, Stool Softner. Also included in many products along with the laxatives **glycerin, casanthranol, bisacodyl,** and **senna.**

Recommended dosage

Highly individualized. The general dose range for adults is 50 to 300 mg a day, but you should follow the manufacturer's recommendations for combination products. Do not take for longer than 1 week. Do not take with **mineral oil** or a prescription drug unless you are under medical supervision.

Side effects and overdosage

Generally well tolerated in recommended doses. May cause nausea, bitter taste, and throat irritation. Skin rashes have been reported.

Synonyms

Docusate calcium, docusate sodium, docusate potassium, dioctyl sodium sulfosuccinate.

Doxylamine

○○○

Use

Antihistamine in the ethanolamine class with significant sedative effects.

Where found

By itself as a sleep aid in Unisom Nighttime Sleep Aid and generics. Also in many cough and cold combinations combined with other ingredients such as **pseudoephedrine, dextromethorphan,** or **acetaminophen** as in Alka-Seltzer Plus Night Time Cold Medicine Liquigels, Clear Cough Night Time, Genite, Night Time Cold Medicine, NiteGel, Robitussin Night-Time Cold Formula, and most Vicks Nyquil products.

Recommended dosage

As a sleep aid: adults and children over 12 years: 25 mg 30 minutes before bedtime. As an antihistamine: adults and children over 12 years: 7.5 to 12.5 mg every 4 to 6 hours, not to exceed 75 mg per day; children 6 to under 12 years: ½ the adult dose; children 2 under 6 years: ¼ the adult dose. Avoid if you are pregnant or nursing.

Side effects and overdosage

Generally well tolerated. As an antihistamine is more sedating than **diphenhydramine.** Some side effects, such as drowsiness, are undesirable when you are taking it during the day and want to stay awake, but desirable when you are taking it to go to sleep. Similarly, a dry nose may be uncomfortable unless you have a cold. Uncommon side effects include allergies, itching, rash, sweating, chills, nervousness, excitability (especially in children), blurred vision, upset stomach, nausea, vomiting, constipation, diarrhea, difficulty with urination, thickening of lung secretions, and wheezing. The sedative effect can be marked with **alcohol,** so avoid this combination. Older people are more sensitive to these side effects. Don't take any antihistamine if you have glaucoma, heart disease, thyroid disease, an enlarged prostate, diabetes, or high blood pressure. Also do not take antihistamines with other sleeping aids, tranquilizers, or antidepressants such as monoamine oxidase inhibitors (MAOIs). Overdosage with doxylamine in addition to other effects has caused severe disruption of heart muscles.

Synonym
Doxylamine succinate.

Dyclonine

○○○

Use
Local anesthetic. Effects last about 30 minutes.

Where found
Orajel CoverMed, Sucrets sore throat lozenges (most), Tanac Medicated Gel.

Recommended dosage
Follow manufacturer's recommendations.

Side effects and overdosage
May cause local irritation.

Synonym
Dyclocaine.

Ephedrine

○○○

Use
Decongestant and asthma reliever. As a decongestant it constricts blood vessels. When taken internally it has stimulant effects similar to **epinephrine,** but less pronounced. Sale is restricted in some states because of its potential for abuse. It is part of the herbal fen-phen formula, along with St. John's wort.

Where found
As a nasal decongestant in Pretz-D nose drops and Quelidrine Cough Syrup. As a hemorrhoidal decongestant in Hydrosal Hemorrhoidal and Pazo. As an asthma reliever in Bronkaid Dual Action Formula, Dynafed Two-Way, Mini Thin Two-Way, and Primatene Tablets. Also has been found in some food supplements and herbal remedies, for example ma huang and Ephedra.

Recommended dosage
For nose drops and hemorrhoid products: follow manufacturer's directions. For asthma relief: adults and children over 12 years: 12.5 to 25 mg every 4 hours, not to exceed 150 mg per day; for children under 12, consult your doctor. Do not use ephedrine unless directed by your doctor. Do not use with any other asthma medications or if you have ever been hospitalized for asthma unless your doctor instructs you to do so. Do not use with the antidepressants known as monoamine oxidase inhibitors (MAOIs) or for 2 weeks after stopping an MAOI. Do not use if you have heart disease, high blood pressure, thyroid disease, diabetes, or an enlarged prostate. If used for asthma and if symptoms are not relieved in 1 hour, call your doctor. Avoid if you are pregnant or nursing.

Side effects and overdosage
May cause rapid or irregular heartbeat, tremor, anxiety, insomnia, nausea, or loss of appetite. Use of nosedrops may cause rebound congestion.

Epinephrine

OOO

Use
Relieves breathing in asthma by opening up the bronchial tubes. Also known as adrenaline, a stimulant hormone produced by the adrenal glands. Medically it is often added to local anesthetics given by injection because it narrows blood vessels, decreases bleeding, and localizes the anesthetic. Its major prescription use, however, is in the control of severe allergic reactions and in cardiac resuscitation and life support.

Where found
As the active ingredient in asthma inhalers such as Asthma-Haler, AsthmaNefrin, Breatheasy, Bronkaid, Epinephrine Mist, microNefrin, and Primatene Mist.

Recommended dosage
Adults and children over 4: 1 inhalation. Repeat in 1 minute if breathing is not relieved. Do not use again for 3 hours. Do not use unless directed by your doctor. Do not use with any other asthma medications or if you have ever been hospitalized for asthma unless your doctor instructs you to do so. Do not use with the antidepressants known as monoamine oxidase inhibitors (MAOIs) or for 2 weeks after stopping an MAOI. Do not use if you have heart disease, high blood pressure, thyroid disease, diabetes, or an enlarged prostate. Avoid if you are pregnant or nursing.

Side effects and overdosage
Usually well tolerated if used as directed. In high doses may cause rapid or irregular heartbeat, tremor, or anxiety.

Synonym
Adrenaline.

Eucalyptol

O O O

Use
Flavoring agent derived from leaves and twigs of various species of *Eucalyptus*. Although sometimes used as a counterirritant in external analgesics, it is not approved by the FDA for this use. Its vapors are aromatic and promote a feeling of refreshing coolness and well being in most individuals.

Where found
Present in numerous sore throat lozenges and Vicks Vapo-Rub, Eucalyptamint, Mentholatum Chest Rub, and Listerine. It is often combined with **menthol** or **camphor.**

Recommended dosage
Follow manufacturer's recommendations.

Side effects and overdosage
May cause irritation to skin and mucous membranes in high doses or strong concentrations.

Synonym
Oil of eucalyptus.

Eugenol

O O O

Use
Topical analgesic derived from cloves. It is the principal ingredient in clove oil. Often mixed with **zinc oxide** and used by dentists in temporary dental fillings.

Where found
Dent-Zel-Ite Toothache Relief and Red Cross Toothache Medication.

Recommended dosage
Use only under the direction of your dentist.

Side effects and overdosage
May cause gum irritation.

Famotidine

OOO

Use
Histamine H_2-receptor antagonist that reduces stomach acid. Approved for prevention and relief of heartburn, indigestion, and sour stomach.

Where found
Mylanta-AR, Pepcid AC.

Recommended dosage
Adults and children over 12 years: For *relief* of symptoms, take 10 mg; if you don't feel better within 1 hour, take another 10 mg. To *prevent* symptoms, take 10 mg 1 hour before eating. Do not exceed 20 mg a day and do not take for longer than 2 weeks.

Side effects and overdosage
Generally well tolerated but may cause headache, dizziness, nausea, and diarrhea.

Ferrous fumarate

OOO

Use
Iron supplement.

Where found
Feostat, Ferro-Sequels, Vitron-C, and others.

Recommended dosage
See **ferrous sulfate** for general recommendations.

Side effects and overdosage
See **ferrous sulfate**.

Ferrous gluconate

○ ○ ○

Use
Iron supplement.

Where found
Fergon, Simron, and others.

Recommended dosage
See **ferrous sulfate** for general guidelines.

Side effects and overdosage
See **ferrous sulfate**.

Ferrous sulfate

○ ○ ○

Use
Iron supplement.

Where found
Feosol, Fer-In-Sol, Mol-Iron, Slow Fe, and many other brand name and generic preparations.

Recommended dosage
The recommended daily allowance for iron is: adults and children over 4: 18 mg; children under 4: 10 mg; infants: 15 mg. The daily dose of ferrous sulfate in adults needed to fulfill this requirement is roughly one 325 mg tablet per day (which contains about 60 mg of iron), but to treat iron

deficiency you need more, usually 325 mg 3 or 4 times a day for 6 months. If treating deficiency, take 1 dose the first day, 2 the second day, and so on until you reach the correct amount. Best if taken on an empty stomach but if it upsets your stomach take it with meals.

Side effects and overdosage
Nausea, diarrhea, and constipation are the most common side effects. Black feces is normal, but may also occur in bleeding from the intestines. Poisoning from excessive iron, especially in children, can result in death. Symptoms of this include nausea, vomiting, diarrhea, abdominal pain, and possibly shock. Ingestion of too much iron over a long time can result in the disease called hemochromatosis, which can cause decreased sex drive, skin pigmentation, liver disease, heart disease, arthritis, and diabetes.

Fluorine

ooo

Use
Nutritional supplement. Fluorine is an element found in bones and teeth combined with calcium as calcium fluoride. The only known symptom of deficiency is excess tooth decay. Those who drink well water or whose water supply is not fluoridated should take supplements.

Where found
Varies widely as a natural substance in soil and water. Most municipal water supplies are fluoridated to increase the amount. Also available topically as **sodium fluoride, sodium monofluorophosphate,** and **stannous fluoride.**

Recommended dosage
Recommended daily allowances (mg): adults and children over 12 years: 1.5 to 4; children: 0.5 to 2.5; infants to 1: 0.1 to 1.

Side effects
Poisoning can occur, deaths having been reported with doses of 500 mg in children and 2 gm in adults. Symptoms of overdose may be abdominal pain, nausea, vomiting, diarrhea, weakness, tremors, and in severe cases seizures. Chronic overuse of fluoride can cause mottling of the teeth and changes in bones.

Folic acid
ooo

Use
Folic acid is a B vitamin with a variety of important biological functions, including a crucial role in DNA synthesis and rapidly dividing cells. Deficiency causes weakness, fatigue, sore mouth, diarrhea, forgetfulness, and irritability. Low folic acid tends to be seen in alcoholism, pregnancy, malabsorption (in which the intestines fail to absorb nutrients properly), malnutrition, and after intestinal bypass surgery. Because vitamin B_{12} is needed for folic acid to work, deficiencies of these two vitamins go together. The main effects of the combined deficiencies are on the blood and nervous system. In the blood, deficiency causes anemia (pernicious anemia) and on the nervous system, nerve damage can result. Only giving folic acid will correct the anemia, but will allow the nerve damage to proceed. This is one reason why it is dangerous to try to treat anemia yourself. Folic acid is especially important in pregnancy and has been shown to prevent the development of neural tube defects, which include spina bifida, in which the bones of the spine do not close properly around the spinal cord, and anencephaly, in which babies are born without brains.

Where found
Meat, dark green leafy vegetables, beans, peas, eggs, grains. Many cereals carry folic acid supplements and it is included in most multivitamins

Recommended dosage

Recommended daily allowances (mcg): adults and children over 4: 400; children under 4: 200; infants: 100; pregnant and nursing women: 800.

Side effects

Large doses are apparently not harmful; toxic effects have not been reported.

Synonyms

Folate, folacin, pteroylglutamic acid.

Glycerin

ooo

Use

Glycerin is a syrupy substance widely employed in the pharmaceutical industry (and in industry in general). Depending upon its concentration it can be a humectant (something that attracts and absorbs water), a demulcent (something that coats and protects mucous membranes), or a protectant, preservative, lubricant, or laxative (hyperosmotic type). As a laxative, some of its effect is produced by irritation of the intestine by sodium stearate in the suppository.

Where found

Vaginal lubricants, nose drops, artificial tears, hemorrhoid products, skin moisturizers, and laxative suppositories.

Recommended dosage

Follow manufacter's recommendations. Avoid glycerin laxative suppositories in pregnancy.

Side effects and overdosage
Rectal irritation is possible from the suppository form. It is toxic if taken orally in large doses and may produce severe dehydration.

Synonym
Glycerol.

Glycolic acid

○ ○ ○

Use
Alpha-hydroxy acid used in cosmetic skin products. Derived from sugar cane.

Where found
Alpha Glow Body Care Lotion and others.

Recommended dosage
Follow manufacturer's recommendations.

Side effects and overdosage
Generally well tolerated but may cause skin irritation.

Guaiacol

○ ○ ○

Use
Counterirritant external analgesic. Formerly it was used as an antiseptic and mucus liquefier (expectorant).

Where found
Methagual (with **methyl salicylate**).

Recommended dosage
Follow manufacturer's recommendations.

Side effects and overdosage
May cause skin irritation.

Guaiafenesin

○○○

Use
Increases and thins mucus in the respiratory tract, but its effectiveness is questionable. Has also been used experimentally to thin cervical mucus in women who were unable to conceive.

Where found
Numerous cough and cold remedies, of which Robitussin is the best known.

Recommended dosage
Adults and children over 12 years: 200 to 400 mg every 4 hours as needed, not to exceed 2400 mg a day. Children 6 to under 12 years: ½ the adult dose. Children 2 to under 6 years: ¼ the adult dose. Do not give to children under 12 if cough is persistent, as in asthma, or if there is excessive mucus. Do not take if you are pregnant unless directed by your doctor.

Side effects and overdosage
Well tolerated but may cause upset stomach in higher than recommended doses. Very large doses can cause vomiting.

Synonym
Glyceryl guaiacolate.

Hard fat

OOO

Use
Protectant in hemorrhoidal suppositories. The name hard fat refers to a large group of fatty substances of different degrees of hardness.

Where found
Anusert, Hem-Prep, Hemorid, Medicone, and Tronolane suppositories.

Recommended dosage
Follow manufacturer's recommendations.

Side effects and overdosage
Well tolerated.

Hexylresorcinol

OOO

Use
Antiseptic. Formerly used internally to kill worms (antihelminthic).

Where found
Various first aid antiseptics and sore throat remedies.

Recommended dosage
Follow manufacturer's recommendations.

Side effects and overdosage
Generally well tolerated in the available OTC preparations, but can cause irritation in higher concentrations.

Homosalate

○ ○ ○

Use
Sunscreen. Tends to be weak and easily removed from the skin by sweating and swimming.

Where found
Coppertone Dry and Tropical Blend Dark Tanning Lotion and Oil (both SPF 2). Also in combination sunscreens.

Recommended dosage
Follow manufacturer's recommendations.

Side effects and overdosage
May cause irritation and sun sensitivity.

Hydrocortisone

○ ○ ○

Use
External anti-inflammatory drug; a hormone secreted by the adrenal cortex and necessary for life. It is the weakest of a large class of topical steroids that are the mainstay of the treatment of inflammatory skin diseases. All other topical steroids are available only by prescription.

Where found
Numerous external dermatitis and anti-itch products in 0.5 to 1 percent concentrations. Prescription strengths are available up to 2.5 percent.

Recommended dosage
Apply 3 times a day as needed and rub in well. Do not use for longer than 7 days. Do not use around the eyes.

Side effects and overdosage
Makes skin infections—such as ringworm, jock itch, athlete's foot, impetigo, yeast, or herpes—worse. There may be

initial improvement but the germ will then flourish. Although absorption of hydrocortisone is negligible under most circumstances, it is possible in some cases, for example in infants when it is applied to the entire skin surface over a prolonged period. If it is applied to thin skin repeatedly for a very long time it may cause thinning of the skin (atrophy), which may show up as a fine wrinkling or increase in superficial blood vessels.

Synonym
Cortisone, cortisol.

Hydrogen peroxide

○ ○ ○

Use
Antiseptic, disinfectant, and deoderant. Used to cleanse wounds, as a bleach, and as a mouthwash. Found in many oral care products and in some contact lens cleaning solutions. It is a very weak antiseptic and its value in wound care, if it has one, is that it cleanses by its effervescent action.

Where found
Many generic sources as a 3 percent solution, and in toothpastes and some contact lens solutions.

Recommended dosage
The 3 percent solution should be applied 1 to 3 times a day to intact skin only.

Side effects and overdosage
Stings on contact with open wounds and may delay healing. Repeated use as a mouthwash can produce enlargement of the tongue papillae and decalcification of the teeth. It is dangerous to drink and to instill hydrogen peroxide into an enclosed body cavity where the oxygen it releases cannot escape. Peroxide enemas have caused rupture of the colon.

274

Hydroquinone

○ ○ ○

Use
Skin lightener for the mask of pregnancy (melasma), freckles, and darkening of the skin from injury. Although it is called a bleach this is not correct. It increases the excretion of melanin from melanocytes and may inhibit its production.

Where found
Ambi, Eldopaque, Eldoquin, Esoterica, Nudit, Palmer's Skin Success, Phade, Porcelana, Solaquin, and Topifram.

Recommended dosage
Apply 2 times a day. Discontinue if irritation develops. Avoid around the eyes.

Side effects and overdosage
Redness, itching, burning, or scaling are possible.

8-Hydroxyquinoline

○ ○ ○

Use
Antiseptic.

Where found
Ammens powder (some), Bagbalm, Burntame (with **benzocaine**), New Skin Liquid Bandage.

Recommended dosage
Follow manufacturer's recommendations.

Side effects and overdosage
Generally well tolerated when used as directed.

Synonym
8-hydroxyquinoline sulfate.

Ibuprofen

○ ○ ○

Use
Reduces pain, inflammation, and fever by interfering with prostaglandins.

Where found
Advil, Dynafed, Haltran, Midol IB Cramp Relief Formula, Motrin, Nuprin, Ultraprin, Valtrin, and generics. Also in several cough and cold combinations.

Recommended dosage
Adults and children over 12 years: 200 to 400 mg every 4 to 6 hours as needed. Do not take more than 1200 mg a day. Children 6 months to under 12 years: 7.5 mg per kg of body weight every 4 to 6 hours as needed, not to exceed 30 mg per kg of body weight a day. Take with food, antacids, or a full glass of water to reduce stomach upset and stomach irritation. Do not take for longer than 10 days for pain or 3 days for fever. Be very careful with **alcohol** intake. If you consume more than 3 drinks a day you probably shouldn't be taking *any* pain reliever. Also, do not take ibuprofen with other pain relievers. Be particularly careful if you are taking blood thinners (anticoagulants) such as warfarin (Coumadin), since the combination can cause serious intestinal bleeding. Ibuprofen may *increase* the effects and toxicity of methotrexate and lithium but may *decrease* the effects of ACE inhibitors (for high blood pressure) and the diuretics furosemide (Lasix) or thiazides (Hydrodiuril). Discontinue for at least 1 day before any type of surgery or dental extraction. Avoid in pregnancy, particularly the last 3 months of pregnancy.

Side effects and overdosage
The most common side effect is upset stomach. The most serious side effect is the production of new stomach ulcers

or the reactivation or perforation of old stomach ulcers. It is particularly important to realize that serious intestinal bleeding (which can be fatal) can occur painlessly and without warning. Although uncommon, life threatening and severe allergic reactions have occurred (anaphylaxis), and those who have a history of asthma, nasal polyps, or angioedema (swelling around the eyes or lips) should be particularly careful. Like other NSAIDs and **aspirin,** ibuprofen may reduce fever sufficiently to give a false sense of security about the severity of an illness. Other side effects are uncommon if ibuprofen is taken as recommended but become more common if the dose or duration of treatment is increased. For example, ibuprofen has been known to cause kidney damage, early signs of which are weakness and loss of appetite. This may be seen particularly in those who are dehydrated, so that adequate fluid intake is important. Liver damage with jaundice is also possible and abnormal liver function tests may occur in as many as 15 percent of those taking NSAIDs. A type of meningitis (aseptic meningitis) has been reported with fever and coma. Visual problems such as blurred vision, decreased visual acuity, and impaired color vision, fluid retention marked by increased weight gain and ankle swelling (shoes feeling tight toward the end of the day), allergic skin rashes, mental confusion, cough, irregular heartbeat, increased blood pressure, and mouth ulcerations are all possible. Signs and symptoms of acute overdosage of NSAIDs may be lethargy, drowsiness, nausea, vomiting, abdominal pain, coma, and convulsions.

Insulin

ooo

Use
Injectable hormone that promotes passage of blood sugar into cells.

Where found
Various products grouped by onset of action into rapid, intermediate, mixed, and long acting.

Recommended dosage
Determined under medical supervision.

Side effects and overdosage
Overdose causes hypoglycemia, which should be treated by administration of sugar.

Iodine
○ ○ ○

Use
1. An element present in the body in trace amounts that is crucial to thyroid function. The symptom of inadequate iodine is the thyroid enlargement known as a goiter. It is very uncommon in the United States. 2. An antiseptic with a broad spectrum of activity.

Where found
Food: iodized table salt, sea salt, saltwater seafood, and vegetables grown in coastal areas. There are two main types of external iodine preparations: iodine tincture is an alcoholic solution of iodine, whereas iodine topical is water based. It is also available as an ointment in Efodine.

Recommended dosage
Recommended daily allowances (mcg): adults and children over 4: 150; children under 4: 70; infants: 45. For external use, apply 2 to 3 times a day.

Side effects and overdosage
Allergies to iodine and iodine compounds are possible whether they are ingested or applied to the skin. Those who ingest large quantities for long periods may develop excess saliva production, sneezing, eye irritation, and a metallic

taste in the mouth. As one increases the amount of iodine in the diet, the activity of the thyroid increases initially but then decreases (hypothyroidism). Avoid the eyes if you are using external products. It may sting if applied to open skin.

Synonym
Sodium iodide.

Ipecac
OOO

Use
To induce vomiting in poisoning. Works by irritating the lining of the stomach and stimulating the nausea centers of the brain. Smaller doses have been employed as expectorants to liquefy sputum and much smaller amounts are sometimes found in homeopathic remedies.

Where found
Syrup of Ipecac (Ipecac Syrup).

Recommended dosage
Always call a Poison Control Center or your doctor first.

Adults and children over 12 years: 15 to 30 ml. Children 1 to under 12 years: 15 ml. Children 6 months to 1: 5 to 10 ml. Should be taken as a single dose with plenty of water or other fluids—children 4 to 8 oz and adults 12 to 16 oz, either before or after the dose. May be repeated if vomiting has not occurred in 20 minutes. The above doses are for Ipecac Syrup only, not for fluidextract of ipecac, which is much stronger. Not useful if the suspected poison has been taken 4 to 6 hours previously. If pregnant, check with your doctor or the Poison Control Center.

Side effects and overdosage
Well tolerated in recommended doses. It is common to have an upset stomach, diarrhea, and mild drowsiness after treatment. Large amounts can cause serious problems by

damaging the heart. Fatalities have been reported in those who have taken large amounts for prolonged periods, as when trying to lose weight.

Kaolin

OOO

Use
Adsorbent in diarrhea control. Also used as a skin protectant and moisture absorbent in hemorrhoidal and diaper rash preparations.

Where found
For diarrhea: generics and Kao-Paverin (along with **pectin** and **bismuth subcarbonate**). Also found in Anusol ointment and some diaper rash products, such as Mexsana Powder (with **zinc oxide, cornstarch,** and **benzethonium chloride**).

Recommended dosage
Follow manufacturer's recommendations. May impair the absorption of other drugs, particularly digitalis (digoxin).

Side effects and overdosage
Very safe but may cause constipation if too much is taken orally.

Synonyms
Aluminum silicate, argilla, China clay, porcelain clay, white bole.

Ketoprofen

OOO

Use
Reduces pain, inflammation, and fever by interfering with prostaglandins.

Where found
Actron, Orudis KT.

Recommended dosage
Adults over 16 years: 12.5 to 25 mg every 4 to 6 hours as needed, not to exceed 75 mg a day. Although food delays absorption of this drug it should be taken with food, antacids, milk, or a full glass of water to reduce stomach upset and stomach irritation. Do not take for longer than 10 days for pain or 3 days for fever. Be very careful with alcohol intake. If you consume more than 3 drinks a day you probably shouldn't be taking *any* pain reliever. Also, do not take with other pain relievers. Be particularly careful if you are taking blood thinners (anticoagulants), since the combination can cause serious intestinal bleeding. Ketoprofen may *increase* the effects and toxicity of methotrexate and lithium but may *decrease* the effects of ACE inhibitors (for high blood pressure) and the diuretics furosemide (Lasix) or thiazides (Hydrodiuril). Discontinue for at least 1 day before any type of surgery or dental extraction. Avoid in pregnancy, particularly the last 3 months.

Side effects and overdosage
The most common side effect is upset stomach. The most serious side effect is the production of new stomach ulcers or the reactivation of old ones. It is particularly important to realize that serious intestinal bleeding can occur painlessly and without warning. Deaths have been reported from such hemorrhage. Although many other side effects are possible, such as allergic skin rashes, mental confusion, cough, irregular heartbeat, increased blood pressure, mouth ulcerations, ankle swelling, weakness, weight gain, and jaundice, most are very uncommon in OTC doses. Side effects tend to be more prounced in women than in men. For other side effects and information about NSAID overdosage, see **ibuprofen.**

Lactase

OOO

Use
Relieves intestinal symptoms in those with lactase deficiency. It is an enzyme that breaks down lactose into glucose and galactose.

Where found
Dairy Ease, Lactaid, Lactrase, SureLac, and generics.

Recommended dosage
For Lactaid add 5 to 7 drops to a quart of milk and refigerate for 24 hours. If symptoms persist, add 10 drops. If you are still having problems, add 15 drops. This amount should remove all the lactose, so if you continue to have intestinal symptoms, see your doctor. May be used with any kind of milk. For other lactase products follow manufacturer's recommendations.

Side effects and overdosage
No reported adverse effects.

Synonym
Beta-d-galactosidase.

Lactic acid

OOO

Use
Alpha-hydroxy skin softening agent added to many cosmetic skin preparations. Aids moisturizers and has some effect in rejuvenating skin damaged by the sun. Formed by fermentation of sugars or produced synthetically. Formerly it was used with **salicylic acid** in wart treatment.

Where found
Lac-Hydrin Five, LactiCare, Soft Sense Alpha Hydroxy Moisturizing Lotion. Also found combined with **urea, malic**

acid, allantoin, or **glycolic acid** in various moisturizers. Concentrations below 10 percent are generally most appropriate for OTC products. Available as a 12 percent lotion by prescription only.

Recommended dosage

Follow manufacturer's recommendations. When used as a moisturizer it is most effective when applied soon after bathing.

Side effects and overdosage

Often stings when first applied. May cause skin irritation if overused.

Lactobacillus acidophilus

OOO

Use

Changes bacteria within the intestine.

Where found

DDS-Acidophilus, Florajen, Probiata, yogurt, and generics.

Recommended dosage

Follow manufacturer's recommendations.

Side effects and overdosage

Well tolerated.

Lanolin

OOO

Use

Moisturizer, protectant, and vehicle for the delivery of medications. It is a fat obtained from wool.

Where found
In many moisturizers, hemorrhoidal products, artificial tear ointments, and diaper rash preparations.

Recommended dosage
Follow manufacturer's recommendations.

Side effects and overdosage
May cause skin irritation. Some individuals who are allergic to one form of lanolin may tolerate purer forms of it.

Lidocaine

○○○

Use
Local anesthetic of the amide type whose duration of action is about 45 minutes. It is by far the most widely used local anesthetic given by injection and is also given intravenously for heart rhythm disturbances.

Where found
Commercially, the brand name Xylocaine is practically synonymous with lidocaine. Most Xylocaine products are available only by prescription, but a 2.5 percent ointment can be purchased OTC. Also found in Bactine First Aid, Banana Boat Sooth-A-Caine, Burn-O-Jel, Burnamycin, Family Medic, Gold Bond Medicated Anti-Itch, Medi-Quik First Aid Spray, Neosporin Plus Maximum Strength, Solarcaine Aloe Extra Burn Relief, Unguentine Plus, and Zilactin-L.

Recommended dosage
Apply 3 to 4 times a day as needed. Do not apply over extensive areas, particularly if the skin is broken.

Side effects and overdosage
Generally very well tolerated. If large amounts are absorbed through the skin—which is very unlikely given the strengths

available and the doses recommended—toxicity in the form of heart and nervous system problems is possible.

Synonym
Lidocaine hydrochloride.

Loperamide

○ ○ ○

Use
Diarrhea control. It is a synthetic relative of opium that works by slowing the movement of the intestine.

Where found
Imodium A-D, Kaodene A-D, Maalox Anti-Diarrheal, Pepto Diarrhea Control, and generics.

Recommended dosage
Adults and children over 12 years: 4 mg initially and 2 mg after each loose bowel movement. Do not take more than 8 mg a day. Children 9 to under 12 years (60 to 95 lb): 2 mg initially and 1 mg after each loose bowel movement. Do not take more than 6 mg a day. Children 6 to under 9 years (48 to 59 lb): 2 mg initially and 1 mg after each loose bowel movement. Do not take more than 4 mg a day. Use in children under 6 is not recommended, but your doctor may suggest loperamide under certain circumstances. In these cases, the guidelines for children 2 to under 6 years (24 to 47 lb) is ½ mg initially and ½ mg after each loose bowel movement, not to exceed 3 mg a day. Do not use if you have liver disease, a tendency to constipation, or inflammatory bowel disease such as ulcerative colitis or Crohn's disease (regional enteritis). Do not use for longer than 2 days or if you have a fever. Do not use if you are taking a narcotic pain killer: severe constipation can result. Tell your doctor if you developed diarrhea while taking an antibiotic.

Side effects
Usually well tolerated but may cause dry mouth, dizziness, fatigue, allergic reactions, constipation, nausea, or vomiting. Large amounts over prolonged periods may cause enlargement of the colon. The symptoms of dehydration, such as dry mouth, hot dry skin, weakness, dizziness, lightheadedness, thirst, and decreased urination may be confused with side effects of loperamide. Large doses in children may result in severe toxic reactions and death.

Synonym
Loperamide hydrochloride.

Magnesium

000

Use
Nutritional supplement. Magnesium is a metallic element important to general metabolism, nerve conduction, and bone structure. Its effects are similar to those of calcium. Magnesium deficiency is uncommon in healthy people on normal diets since magnesium is so widespread in foods. But it is sometimes seen in those with intestinal malabsorption (in which there is failure to absorb nutrients properly) or when increased amounts are excreted, as might occur in kidney disease, with certain medications, and chronic diarrhea. Magnesium deficiency sometimes occurs also in alcoholics. Symptoms of deficiency include depression, irregular heart beat, muscle twitching, and muscle cramps. Severe deficiency may lead to convulsions.

Where found
Unprocessed vegetables, particularly nuts, seeds, beans, grains, green vegetables, and nutritional supplements.

Recommended dosage
Recommended daily allowance (mg): adult males: 350; adult females: 280. Increase by 20 mg in pregnancy and 75 mg when nursing.

Side effects and overdosage

Magnesium toxicity may result in mental confusion, muscle weakness, nausea, vomiting, heart rhythm irregularities, and shock. Be extremely careful with magnesium supplements if you have kidney disease. Magnesium sulfate and magnesium hydroxide taken for laxative or antacid effects may cause magnesium toxicity in those with kidney disease, but healthy people will excrete the excess.

Synonym

Magnesium gluconate.

Magnesium carbonate

o o o

Use

Antacid that reacts with stomach (hydrochloric) acid to form magnesium chloride and carbon dioxide gas.

Where found

Various antacids (see Chapter 16), usually combined with ingredients containing aluminum.

Recommended dosage

Follow manufacturer's recommendations. In general it is best to allow 1 or 2 hours to elapse between taking antacids and taking other medications. In the case of ciprofloxacin (Cipro) and other quinolone antibiotics, antacids should be taken at least 6 hours before or 2 hours after the antibiotic. Many drug interactions are possible.

Side effects and overdosage

May cause diarrhea and excessive gas (flatulence and belching) because of the carbon dioxide produced.

Magnesium citrate

OOO

Use
Saline type laxative. Works by drawing water into the intestine, increasing volume, and stimulating evacuation. Works in 30 minutes to 3 hours. Used for rapid emptying of the bowel before certain medical tests or as a purge for poisons.

Where found
Evac-Q-Kwik liquid, generics.

Recommended dosage
Adults and children over 12 years: 240 mL. Children: 0.5 mL per kg, but check with your doctor first. Do not use for longer than 1 week. Avoid in pregnancy.

Side effects and overdosage
Significant **magnesium** may be absorbed if used for prolonged periods, creating **magnesium** toxicity (see under **magnesium**). Also may cause dehydration by causing the elimination of fluid.

Magnesium hydroxide

OOO

Use
Antacid and laxative. As a laxative it generally acts in 30 minutes to 3 hours. Sometimes used as a magnesium supplement and may be used as a food additive.

Where found
Phillips' Milk of Magnesia is the most well known preparation. It is also found in Creamalin, Haleys M-O, Maalox (some), Mylanta (some), Tempo drops, and generics.

Recommended dosage

Follow manufacturer's recommendations. In small doses, up to about 1 gm, it functions as an antacid. But slightly higher amounts, up to about 5 gm, have a laxative effect. Avoid in pregnancy. In general it is best to allow 1 or 2 hours to elapse between taking antacids and taking other medications. In the case of ciprofloxacin (Cipro) and other quinolone antibiotics, antacids should be taken at least 6 hours before or 2 hours after the antibiotic. Many drug interactions are possible.

Side effects and overdosage

Large amounts may cause **magnesium** toxicity (see under **magnesium**).

Magnesium oxide

OOO

Use

Antacid, laxative, and **magnesium** source. It is converted to **magnesium hydroxide** in water.

Where found

Mag-Ox 400, Uro-Mag, and many vitamin and mineral products.

Recommended dosage

Follow manufacturer's recommendations.

Side effects and overdosage

See **magnesium**.

Magnesium salicylate

OOO

Use

Reduces pain, fever, and inflammation.

Where found
Doan's products and generics usually labelled for backache. Also in Arthriten, Backache From the Makers of Nuprin, Mobigesic, and Momentum.

Recommended dosage
Adults: 377 to 754 mg every 4 hours as needed, not to exceed 4640 mg a day. Do not give to children or teenagers 15 years of age or younger with flu or chickenpox symptoms. Be careful when taking with other salicylates, such as **aspirin** or **bismuth subsalicylate** or with foods high in salicylates, such as raisins, licorice, prunes, or tea. Do not take with other pain relievers, blood thinners, or methotrexate. Do not use if you have kidney disease. Avoid in pregnancy, particularly the last 3 months.

Side effects and overdosage
See **aspirin**. Generally well tolerated in recommended doses. Higher doses may cause ringing in the ears and dizziness.

Synonym
Magnesium salicylate tetrahydrate.

Magnesium stearate
○ ○ ○

Use
Moisture absorber in powders. May also be found in some creams and tablets.

Where found
ZBT Baby Powder (with **talc**).

Recommended dosage
Follow manufacturer's recommendations. Avoid inhaling powder.

Side effects and overdosage
Well tolerated when used as directed.

Magnesium sulfate

OOO

Use
Saline type laxative. Works by drawing water into the intestine, increasing volume, and stimulating evacuation. Works in 30 minutes to 3 hours. Used for rapid emptying of the bowel before certain medical tests or as a purge for poisons.

Where found
Epsom salt and Metamucil Smooth Sugar-Free, Regular Flavor (with **psyllium**).

Recommended dosage
Variable and should be individualized. The general range for adults and children over 12 years is 10 to 30 gm a day. For children 6 to under 12 years it is 5 to 10 gm a day, and for children 2 to under 6 years it is 2.5 to 5 gm a day. Take each dose with at least 8 oz of water or other fluid. Do not use for longer than 1 week.

Side effects and overdosage
Significant **magnesium** may be absorbed if used for prolonged periods, creating **magnesium** toxicity. Also may cause dehydration by causing the elimination of fluid.

Magnesium trisilicate

OOO

Use
Antacid. Reacts slowly with stomach (hydrochloric) acid to produce magnesium chloride and silicon dioxide, which are then excreted. It may react so slowly that little neutralizing of acid has occurred before it passes out of the stomach. It is also sometimes used as a food additive.

Where found

Gaviscon-2 tablets (with **aluminum hydroxide, sodium bicarbonate,** and **alginic acid**) and XS Hangover Relief (with **calcium carbonate, calcium citrate, acetaminophen,** and **caffeine**).

Recommended dosage

Follow manufacturer's guidelines. May be given in doses up to about 2 gm. In general it is best to allow 1 or 2 hours to elapse between taking antacids and taking other medications. In the case of ciprofloxacin (Cipro) and other quinolone antibiotics, antacids should be taken at least 6 hours before or 2 hours after the antibiotic. Many drug interactions are possible.

Side effects and overdosage

See **magnesium**.

Malic acid

ooo

Use

Alpha-hydroxy skin softening agent derived from apples, pears, and other fruits. Sometimes used as a food additive.

Where found

Neutraderm 30 (with **lactic acid, petrolatum, silicone,** and **glycerin**).

Recommended dosage

Follow manufacturer's recommendations.

Side effects and overdosage

Usually well tolerated but may cause irritation.

Malt soup extract

○ ○ ○

Use
Laxative in the bulk forming class derived from barley malt (sometimes with a small amount of wheat malt). Also tends to make the feces more acidic, which may contribute to its laxative effect. Usually works in 12 to 24 hours but may take as long as 3 days. Has nutritional value in that it contains carbohydrates and protein.

Where found
Maltsupex powder, liquid, and tablets.

Recommended dosage
Adult and children over 12 years: 4 tablets (3 gm) 4 times a day. This dose may be increased as needed but do not take more than 48 tablets a day. For the powder and liquid forms see manufacturer's guidelines and take the smallest dose that works. Doses are given for corrective and maintenance of bowel function. The corrective (larger) doses are designed for 3 to 4 days. Ranges are given for infants over one month to adults. Do not use for longer than one week. Take each dose with adequate fluid: at least 8 oz of water, fruit juice, or other liquids.

Side effects and overdosage
As with all bulk forming laxatives, the most serious side effect is blockage of the esophagus (the food tube that leads from the throat to the stomach) or choking if not enough fluid is taken with the product. Note manufacturer's estimate of sodium content if you are on a low sodium diet and the carbohydrate content if you are diabetic.

Synonym
Malt extract.

Manganese

○ ○ ○

Use
Nutritional supplement (elemental metal). Although found in small amounts it is essential to the proper functioning of many enzymes in the body. Deficiency is extremely rare—only one case has ever been reported, in which there was nausea, vomiting, weight loss, and changes in the hair and nails. There is no reason to take supplements.

Where found
Widely found in vegetables, fruits, nuts, beans, peas, grains, coffee, tea, and nutritional supplements.

Recommended dosage
Recommended daily allowance (mg): adults and children 11 and over: 2.5 to 5; children 7 to 10: 2 to 3; children 4 to 6: 1.5 to 2; children 1 to 3: 1 to 1.5; 6 mos to 1 year: 0.7 to 1; infancy to 6 months: 0.5–0.7.

Side effects and overdosage
Manganese toxicity may cause nausea, vomiting, headache, psychiatric, and nervous disturbances. This can occur in industrial exposure and after liver transplantation (due to decreased excretion). Some water supplies are contaminated with it. The nervous system abnormalties may be permanent.

Meclizine

○ ○ ○

Use
An antihistamine that acts to prevent motion sickness. It may work by blocking certain receptor sites in the brain or by depressing nerve impulses in the ear. It is a member of the piperazine class of antihistamines, like **cyclizine,** but is longer acting (12 to 24 hours).

Where found
Bonine and Dramamine II.

Recommended dosage
Adults and children over 12 years: 25 to 50 mg one hour before travel, not to exceed 50 mg a day. Chewable tablets are available (Bonine). Not recommended for children under 12. Avoid if you are pregnant or nursing.

Side effects and overdosage
Generally well tolerated with less sedation than some other histamines. Besides drowsiness, dryness of the nose and mouth is relatively common. Uncommon side effects include allergies, itching, rash, sweating, chills, nervousness, excitability (especially in children), blurred vision, upset stomach, nausea, vomiting, constipation, diarrhea, difficulty with urination, thickening of lung secretions, and wheezing. The sedative effect can be marked with **alcohol,** so avoid this combination. Older people are more sensitive to these side effects. Don't take any antihistamine if you have glaucoma, thyroid disease, an enlarged prostate, diabetes, or high blood pressure. Also do not take antihistamines with other sleeping aids, tranquilizers, or antidepressants such as monoamine oxidase inhibitors (MAOIs). For lung diseases such as asthma, emphysema, or chronic bronchitis, check with your doctor.

Melatonin

o o o

Use
Sleep aid and for reducing jet lag. It is a hormone naturally found in the pineal gland.

Where found
Melatonex (with **vitamin B₆**) and generics. Pills and a spray form are available.

Recommended dosage

The best dose is not known. Most manufacturers recommend 3 to 9 mg as needed for sleep, not to exceed 9 mg a day, but this is probably too high. The experimental dose for reducing jet lag is 5 mg at night for one week, starting three days before the flight. Do not take if you are pregnant or nursing. Do not take unless you are under medical supervision.

Side effects and overdosage

May cause excessive drowsiness and a hangover. May also cause breast enlargement and diminished reproductive capacity.

Menthol

OOO

Use

Flavoring agent, nasal decongestant, topical cough suppressant, external anti-itch ingredient, and counterirritant. The effect is generally related to its strength. When applied to the skin, menthol produces a cool sensation followed by a warm sensation. The effect is to confuse the nerve endings, masking pain and itching. Most people like the scent and taste, and the placebo effect is significant. The name comes from Mentha, the genus that includes various mints. Menthol is related to camphor, but not so toxic. It has also been employed in the past as a carminative (something that reduces intestinal gas and intestinal movement), but this use is not approved by the FDA.

Where found

Very widely distributed in candy, cough drops, chewing gum, toothpaste, and nasal sprays. In external analgesics it is found in products such as Absorbine jr., BenGay, Blistex, Chap Stick, Mentholatum, Icy Hot, Noxzema, Vicks Vapo-Rub, Wonder Ice, generics, and many others. In anti-itch preparations it is found in such products such as Gold Bond Powder, Sarna Lotion, Rhuli, and others. Most often used in combination with other ingredients.

Recommended dosage
Follow manufacturer's directions.

Side effects and overdosage
In view of its almost universal distribution, the rate of side effects is probably very low, although deaths have occurred from ingestion of large amounts. Heart rhythm disturbances (arrhythmias) have also been reported. Some individuals are allergic to it and may develop rashes, hives, and breathing problems. It has also been known to trigger attacks of asthma. Cases of irritation of the lips have been traced to the menthol in toothpaste.

Synonyms
Peppermint oil, peppermint camphor.

Menthyl anthranilate

○ ○ ○

Use
Sunscreen. Tends to be weak, but good for UVA.

Where found
Usually formulated in combination with UVB sunscreens.

Recommended dosage
Follow manufacturer's recommendations.

Side effects and overdosage
May cause irritation and sun sensitivity.

Merbromin

○ ○ ○

Use
A feeble antiseptic which is a combination of mercury and the dye fluorescein.

Where found
Mercurochrome.

Recommended dosage
Follow manufacturer's directions. Since there are better antiseptic alternatives, the use of this product is not recommended.

Side effects and overdosage
Well tolerated.

Methyl nicotinate

ooo

Use
A counterirritant in external analgesics that dilates blood vessels and reddens the skin.

Where found
ArthriCare Pain Relieving Rub (with **menthol** and **capsaicin**) and ArthriCare Triple Medicated Pain Relieving Rub (with **menthol** and **methyl salicylate**).

Recommended dosage
Adults and children over 2 years: apply 3 to 4 times a day as needed. Do not use in children under 2.

Side effects and overdosage
In recommended doses it is well tolerated. High concentrations applied over large areas may produce a drop in blood pressure.

Methyl salicylate

ooo

Use
Widely used counterirritant in external analgesics and flavoring agent in many products.

Where found

External analgesics: ArthriCare Triple Medicated Pain Relieving Rub, Arthritis Hot, Arthritis Rub Extra Strength, Banalg Muscle Pain Reliever, many BenGay products, Gold Bond products, Heet, Icy Hot, Mentholatum products, plus others and generics. Available as lotions, creams, ointments, gels, and powders. Much smaller concentrations are used in flavorings.

Recommended dosage

Adults over the age of 15 years: apply 3 to 4 times a day as needed. Do not cover with a tight bandage and do not apply heat. Avoid if you are pregnant or breast feeding. Do not apply to children or teenagers under the age of 15 with symptoms of flu or chickenpox. Do not use for longer than 7 days unless directed by your doctor.

Side effects and overdosage

In recommended concentrations and use, it is well tolerated. If used with a heating pad, however, skin ulcers down to the muscle have occured. Do not apply immediately after exercise, if you are overheated, or if you are in a hot environment because absorption through the skin will be greatly increased. This preparation is a salicylate related to **aspirin** and is easily absorbed through the skin so that precautions in those who are sensitive to salicylates are warranted. Large amounts taken orally have caused death in infants and children.

Synonyms

Oil of wintergreen, checkerberry oil, sweet birch oil, gaultheria oil, teaberry oil.

Methylbenzethonium chloride

ooo

Use

Antiseptic in the quaternary ammonium class.

Where found
Diapa-Kare Powder.

Recommended dosage
Follow manufacturer's recommendations.

Side effects and overdosage
May cause skin irritation.

Methylcellulose

ooo

Use
Bulk forming laxative derived from synthetic cellulose. Usually works in 12 to 24 hours but may take as long as 3 days. Methylcellulose itself is widely used in drug manufacturing to thicken liquid suspensions and creams.

Where found
Citrucel.

Recommended dosage
Adults and children over 12 years: 2 gm 1 to 3 times a day as needed. Do not take more than 6 gm a day. One rounded tablespoon of Citrucel, which is approximately 19 gm, contains 2 gm of methylcellulose. Must be mixed and taken with at least 8 oz of water, fruit juice, soda, or other liquid. More liquid is even better. Do not use for longer than 1 week.

Side effects and overdosage
The most serious side effect is blockage of the esophagus or choking if not enough fluid is taken.

Miconazole

○○○

Use
External treatment of fungus and yeast infections, such as ringworm, athlete's foot, jock itch, vaginal yeast or sun fungus (tinea versicolor).

Where found
Absorbine jr. (some), Breezee Mist, Desenex AF, Fungoid Tincture, Lotrimin (some), Micatin, Tetterine, and Zeasorb-AF. Vaginal yeast products: Monistat 7, Yeast-X. Available as aerosols, creams, lotions, solutions, and powders.

Recommended dosage
Apply 2 times a day and follow manufacturer's recommendations. Keep away from your eyes. OTC antifungal products are not designed for scalp ringworm.

Side effects
Allergies are uncommon. Discontinue if you experience increased redness, blisters, or a burning sensation.

Mineral oil

○○○

Use
Widely used as a vehicle for the delivery of medications and in many skin moisturizers. Also used in artificial tear ointments and as a protectant in hemorrhoidal preparations. Can be used as a lubricant laxative and stool softener that works by keeping feces moist. For this purpose it usually works in 6 to 8 hours. Comes in light and heavy forms.

Where found

As a vehicle and protectant it is found in many skin, hemorrhoid, and eye products. As a laxative it is in Fleet Mineral Oil Oral Lubricant, Fleet Mineral Oil Enema, Kondremul, Liqui-Doss, Milkinol, and generics. Also may be found combined with **magnesium hydroxide** in Haleys M-O.

Recommended dosage

Laxative use: Highly individual. The dose range in adults is one to three tablespoons (15 to 45 ml) a day as needed. Do not lie down immediately afterward. The last dose should be taken 2 hours before dinner so that food washes the substance out of the stomach before bedtime. In children over 6 the range is two to three teaspoons (10 to 15 ml) a day. Avoid if you are pregnant. Do not take within 2 hours of meals because of possible interference with digestion and absorption of foods. Do not take for longer than 1 week. Do not take with the stool softener **docusate** nor with with oral anticoagulants (blood thinners) such as warfarin (Coumadin). For other uses follow manufacturer's recommendations.

Side effects and overdosage

Generally well tolerated in external preparations. When used as a laxative, however, it has caused aspiration into the lungs causing pneumonia, a complication that is promoted by lying flat after taking an oral dose. Prolonged use interferes with the absorption of the fat soluble vitamins A, D, E, and K. In general, mineral oil for laxative use is best avoided. There are better laxatives and stool softeners.

Synonym

Liquid petrolatum, liquid paraffin, paraffin oil.

Minoxidil

OOO

Use

Hair regrower for common (male pattern or androgenetic) baldness. Used in prescription form, rarely, as a powerful drug for high blood pressure.

Where found
Consort, HealthGuard Minoxidil, Rogaine, and generics.

Recommended dosage
Adults over the age of 18 years: apply 2 times a day, indefinitely. Follow the instructions in the package regarding the use and choice of applicators. If you haven't seen results in a year you should abandon treatment. Do not use if your hair loss is sudden or patchy, if your scalp is inflamed, or if you do not know the reason for your hair loss. Discontinue if you experience chest pain, headache, rapid heartbeat, faintness, dizziness, unexplained weight gain, swelling of the hands or feet, or skin irritation.

Side effects and overdosage
Generally well tolerated, but may cause itching, stinging, burning, or other skin irritation. Unwanted hair growth on other parts of the body has been reported.

Molybdenum

OOO

Use
Nutritional supplement. Although this trace element is important for the proper functioning of several enzyme systems in the body, diseases caused by its deficiency or excess are very rare.

Where found
Peas, beans, grains, liver, kidney, dark green vegetables, and nutritional supplements.

Recommended dosage
Recommended daily allowance (mg): adults and children over 11: 0.15–0.5; children 7 to 10: 0.1–0.3; children 4 to 6: 0.06–0.15; 1 to 3: 0.05–0.1; 6 m–1 year: 0.04–0.08; birth to 1: 0.03–0.06.

Side effects and overdosage
Molybenum toxicity may produce liver disease, kidney disease, and arthritis. Overexposure may occur in certain industries or in certain geographical locations with a high soil content of the element.

Mustard oil
ooo

Use
Externally applied analgesic and counterirritant. It was formerly a popular home remedy mixed with an adhesive, such as flour and lukewarm water, and applied as a mustard plaster to a paper or cotton cloth.

Where found
Numol (with methyl salicylate, camphor, and menthol).

Recommended dosage
Adults and children over 2: Apply 3 to 4 times a day. Do not use for longer than 7 days.

Side effects and overdosage
Mustard oil typically reddens the skin and makes it feel hot. In the case of a typical mustard plaster this occurs within about 5 minutes. If left on longer than 15 to 30 minutes blisters can form. In high concentrations mustard oil is rapidly absorbed from the skin and can be highly irritating, with the potential for skin ulcers. Undiluted it is a toxic substance and *should not be inhaled or ingested.* The presently available commercial product, however, contains a dilute amount and should have a low rate of complications.

Synonyms
Allyl isothiocyanate, essence of mustard.

Naphazoline

ooo

Use

Short acting topical nasal and eye decongestant that works by narrowing blood vessels. Such drugs are known as vasoconstrictors.

Where found

As a nasal decongestant in 4-Way (with **pyrilamine**) and Privine. Found in many eye drops, such as 20/20, Allerest, Clear Eyes products, Estivin II, Naphcon, OcuHist, Opcon-A, Sensitive Eyes Redness Reliever Lubricant, Vaso Clear, and Vasocon-A.

Recommended dosage

Nasal decongestant, 0.05 percent solution: adults and children over 12 years: 1 to 2 drops or sprays every 6 hours as needed. Not for children under 12. The 0.025 percent solution can be used in the same dose for adults and children over 6. Eye drops: follow manufacturer's directions. Usually it is 1 to 2 drops in the affected eyes up to 4 times a day. If you have glaucoma, check with your doctor. Do not use either kind of preparation for more than 3 days. Avoid if you are pregnant or nursing. Do not use if you have heart disease, high blood pressure, thyroid disease, diabetes, or an enlarged prostate

Side effects and overdosage

Nasal products may cause burning, stinging, sneezing, increased nasal discharge, and irritation. Eye products may produce eye pain, blurry vision, and irritation, as well as enlargement of the pupil. Rebound congestion may occur, in which reflex widening (dilatation) of blood vessels causes persistent nasal stuffiness or eye redness despite ever-increasing doses.

Naproxen

ooo

Use
Reduces pain, inflammation, and fever by interfering with
prostaglandins.

Where found
Aleve.

Recommended dosage
Adults under 65 years and over 12 years: 220 to 440 mg
every 8 to 12 hours as needed, not to exceed 660 mg a day.
Adults over 65 years: 220 mg every 12 hours as needed, not
to exceed 440 mg a day. Take with food, antacids, or a full
glass of water to reduce stomach upset and stomach irritation. Do not take for longer than 10 days for pain or 3 days
for fever. Be very careful with alcohol intake. If you
consume more than 3 drinks a day you probably shouldn't
be taking *any* pain reliever. Also, do not take with other
pain relievers. Be particularly careful if you are taking
blood thinners (anticoagulants), since the combination can
cause serious intestinal bleeding. Naproxen may *increase*
the effects and toxicity of methotrexate and lithium but may
decrease the effects of ACE inhibitors (for high blood
pressure) and the diuretics furosemide (Lasix) or thiazides
(Hydrodiuril). Discontinue for at least 1 day before any type
of surgery or dental extraction. Avoid in pregnancy, particularly the last 3 months.

Side effects and overdosage
The most common side effect is upset stomach. The most
serious side effect is the production of new stomach ulcers
or the reactivation of old ones. It is particularly important
to realize that serious bleeding can occur painlessly and
without warning. Deaths have been reported from such
hemorrhage. Although many other side effects are possible,
such as allergic skin rashes, mental confusion, cough, irregular heartbeat, increased blood pressure, mouth ulcerations, ankle swelling, weakness, weight gain, and jaundice,

most are very uncommon. For other side effects and information about NSAID overdosage, see **ibuprofen.**

Neomycin

OOO

Use
Broad spectrum antibiotic whose use is now mostly confined to external applications because of toxicity when taken internally.

Where found
Myciguent and generics. With **bacitracin** and **polymyxin B** in various triple antibiotics such as Campho-phenique Triple Antibiotic, Clomycin, Lanabiotic, Mycitracin, Neosporin, and Tri-Biozene.

Recommended dosage
Apply 1 to 3 times a day.

Side effects and overdosage
Generally well tolerated when applied to small areas of intact skin, but about 5 percent of people are allergic to it and develop significant skin irritation. If applied in very large amounts to wide areas of broken skin it may be absorbed and produce ear and kidney damage.

Niacin

OOO

Use
Niacin is a vitamin essential to the proper functioning of every cell in the body. The classic niacin deficiency state is called pellagra, the symptoms of which are the 3 Ds: diarrhea, dermatitis (skin rash), and dementia. Deficiency is usually associated with malnutrition or alcoholism. Niacin in higher than recommended amounts (about 1000 mg a

day) helps lower cholesterol and triglycerides and has been used to lower these blood fats. It also increases the HDL (good cholesterol) and decreases LDL (bad cholesterol), but it is not widely used because of its numerous side effects.

Where found
Meats, fish, grains, green vegetables, eggs, nuts, beans, peas, and nutritional supplements. About half the body's supply comes from the conversion of the amino acid tryptophan, present in many proteins.

Recommended dosage
Recommended daily allowances (mg): adults and children over 4: 20; children under 4: 9; infants: 8; pregnant and nursing women: 20.

Side effects and overdosage
High doses cause flushing and burning sensations of the skin, and can produce nausea, vomiting, diarrhea, rapid heart rate, high blood pressure, and liver damage. Niacin can worsen ulcers, gastritis, asthma, diabetes, liver disease, or gout. Doses of higher than 500 mg per day should not be taken without medical supervision.

Synonym
Nicotinic acid, nicotinamide, vitamin B_3.

Nicotine

OOO

Use
As a drug, nicotine is usually classified as a ganglionic stimulant, a ganglion being a collection of nerve endings. With large doses, however, the stimulation turns into paralysis. As an OTC product, nicotine is used to help quit tobacco use.

Where found
Nicoderm CQ, Nicorette, Nicotrol. (Nicorette is chewing gum. Nicoderm and Nicotrol are patches).

Recommended dosage

Nicorette comes in 2 mg and 4 mg doses, the larger being for those who smoke more than 24 cigarettes a day. The following is the general schedule: 2 to 4 mg every 1 to 2 hours for the first 6 weeks; 2 to 4 mg every 2 to 4 hours for the next 3 weeks; 2 to 4 mg every 4 to 8 hours for the final 3 weeks.

Nicoderm CQ comes as patches with 7 mg, 14 mg, or 21 mg of nicotine. The schedule for healthy people is: 21 mg a day for the first 6 weeks; 14 mg a day for the next 2 weeks; 7 mg a day for the final 2 weeks.

Nicotrol comes as a single dose patch of 15 mg. The recommended regimen is to apply one patch during waking hours for 6 weeks.

Do not use any of these if you still smoke cigarettes, cigars, or a pipe, chew tobacco, or use snuff. Be careful if you have high blood pressure, heart disease, ulcers or other digestive problems, thyroid disease, diabetes, or take medications for asthma or depression. Discontinue if you develop a rapid or irregular heartbeat or palpitations. Do not apply to broken skin. Avoid if you are pregnant or nursing.

Side effects and overdosage

May cause nausea, vomiting, dizziness, weakness, or irregular heartbeat. Patches may cause local skin irritation. This can be reduced by rotating the site of patch application. Nicotine (and smoking) tends to decrease the effects of analgesics such as **acetaminophen, aspirin, ibuprofen, ketoprofen,** and **naproxen** and of heartburn medications such as **cimetidine, famotidine,** and **ranitidine.** It also decreases the effects of certain anticoagulants (blood thinners), diuretics (water pills), high blood pressure medications, heart medications, antidepressants, and **vitamin C.** There have been reports of heart attacks and strokes occurring in those wearing nicotine patches, but it is not known if the patches were the cause.

Nizatidine

○○○

Use
Reduces stomach acid by blocking histamine₂ receptors. Used to prevent and treat heartburn, indigestion, and sour stomach.

Where found
Axid AR.

Recommended dosage
Adults and children over 12 years: take 75 mg 2 times a day as needed. Although not currently labelled "for relief," 75 mg may be taken when symptoms occur. Do not take more than 150 mg a day or for longer than 2 weeks. Prescription doses can be as high as 300 mg per day when used to treat stomach ulcers or severe inflammation of the esophagus.

Side effects and overdosage
Generally well tolerated but may cause anemia and allergic reactions. In men, there have been reports of excessive sweating, impotence, and enlargement of the breasts.

Nonoxynol-9

○○○

Use
Spermicide, antiseptic, and surface active agent (detergent).

Where found
Numerous contraceptive foams, jellies, creams, suppositories, films, and condoms, such as Advantage 24, CarePlus, Conceptrol, Delfen, Emko, Encare, Gynol II, K-Y Plus, Koromex, Ortho-Creme, Ortho-Gynol, Semicid, Shur-Seal, and VCF.

Recommended dosage
Follow manufacturer's recommendations.

Side effects and overdosage
Generally well tolerated but may cause local irritation.

Oatmeal

OOO

Use
Skin protectant. Hydrating and soothing agent.

Where found
As colloidal oatmeal in Aveeno products and other skin moisturizers.

Recommended dosage
Follow manufacturer's recommendations.

Side effects and overdosage
Safe.

Octocrylene

OOO

Use
Sunscreen with broad range in both UVB and UVA. Tends not to stick well to the skin.

Where found
Many combination sunscreens.

Recommended dosage
Follow manufacturer's recommendations.

Side effects and overdosage
May cause irritation and sun sensitivity.

Octoxynol-9

O O O

Use
Spermicide.

Where found
Ortho-Gynol Jelly.

Recommended dosage
Follow manufacturer's recommendations. This product is designed to be used with a diaphragm.

Side effects and overdosage
Generally well tolerated.

Octyl methoxycinnamate

O O O

Use
Sunscreen effective against UVB. Tends not to stick well to the skin.

Where found
In combination with other sunscreens.

Recommended dosage
Follow manufacturer's recommendations.

Side effects and overdosage
May cause irritation and sun sensitivity.

Octyl salicylate

O O O

Use
Sunscreen effective against UVB, as are other salicylate sunscreens. Tends to be weak and easily removed from the skin by sweating and swimming.

Where found
Several combination sunscreens.

Recommended dosage
Follow manufacturer's recommendations.

Side effects and overdosage
May cause irritation and sun sensitivity.

Oil of citronella

O O O

Use
Insect repellent. An old remedy, popular during World War II, but much less effective than DEET.

Where found
Avon Skin So Soft, Natrapel, Green Ban, ZZZ Away, Treo.

Recommended dosage
Follow manufacturer's recommendations.

Side effects and overdosage
Generally safe when used as directed.

Oxybenzone

O O O

Use
Sunscreen with both UVA and UVB activity.

Where found
Usually combined with other sunscreens for broader range of coverage.

Recommended dosage
Follow manufacturer's recommendations.

Side effects and overdosage
May cause irritation and sun sensitivity.

Oxymetazoline

○ ○ ○

Use
Long acting decongestant in nasal sprays and eye drops.
Works by narrowing blood vessels. Such drugs are called
vasoconstrictors.

Where found
In nasal decongestants it is found in 4-Way Long Lasting,
Afrin products (most), Cheracol, Dristan 12-Hour, Dura-
tion, Neo-Synephrine 12 Hour, and Vicks Sinex 12-Hour.
In eye products it is in OcuClear and Visine L.R.

Recommended dosage
Nasal 0.05 percent solution: adults and children over 6
years: 2 to 3 drops or sprays every 12 hours as needed.
Nasal 0.025 percent solution: adults and children over 2
years: 2 to 3 drops or sprays every 12 hours as needed. Eye
0.025 percent solution: adults and children over 6: 1 or 2
drops in the affected eyes every 6 hours as needed. Do not
use for more than 3 days. Do not use if you have heart
disease, high blood pressure, thyroid disease, diabetes,
glaucoma, or an enlarged prostate. Avoid if you are pregnant or nursing.

Side effects and overdosage
Nasal products may cause burning, stinging, sneezing, increased nasal discharge, and irritation. Rebound congestion, in which reflex dilatation of blood vessels causes
persistant nasal stuffiness despite ever increasing doses may
occur but is less common with oxymetazoline than it is with
other topical nasal decongestants because it is longer acting.
Eye products may produce eye pain, blurry vision, irrita-

tion, or rebound redness. In this case, however, oxymetazo-line may produce *greater* rebound redness than **naphazoline** or **tetrahydrozoline.**

Oxyquinoline

○ ○ ○

Use
Antiseptic.

Where found
Trimo-San Jelly.

Recommended dosage
Follow manufacturer's recommendations.

Side effects and overdosage
Generally well tolerated when used as directed.

Synonym
Oxyquinoline sulfate.

Padimate O

○ ○ ○

Use
Sunscreen, derivative of PABA. Penetrates skin well and resists sweating.

Where found
Mentholatum Lipbalm, Softlips Crystal Ice and Sparkle Mint, and many combination sunscreens.

Recommended dosage
Follow manufacturer's recommendations.

Side effects and overdosage
May cause irritation and sun sensitivity.

Pamabrom

OOO

Use
Promotes fluid excretion (diuretic) and relieves menstrual discomfort. It is related chemically to **caffeine.**

Where found
Aqua-Ban and Odrinil Water Pills. Also in combination products along with **acetaminophen** in Backaid Pills, Bayer Select Aspirin-Free Menstrual, Diurex products (most), Fem-1, Lurline PMS, Midol products (most), Pamprin products, and Premsyn PMS.

Recommended dosage
Adults and children over 12 years: 50 mg every 4 to 6 hours as needed, not to exceed 200 mg per day. Do not use for longer than 10 days.

Side effects and overdosage
No reported adverse effects in recommended doses.

Pancreatin

OOO

Use
A mixture of three pancreatic digestive enzymes used in the treatment of cystic fibrosis and other diseases of the pancreas. Amylase breaks starch down into maltose; lipase breaks fat down into fatty acids and **glycerin;** protease (trypsin) breaks proteins down into peptides.

Where found
Several OTC and prescription products.

Recommended dosage
Follow manufacturer's recommendations, but use only under a doctor's supervision.

Side effects and overdosage
May have a laxative effect if too much is taken.

Pantothenic acid

OOO

Use
Pantothenic acid is a water soluble vitamin important to general metabolism. When deficiency occurs, which is very rare, it is usually part of a general malnutrition with other vitamin deficiencies. Symptoms of deficiency include fatigue, headache, and tingling of the hands and feet.

Where found
Widely distributed in many foods.

Recommended dosage
Recommended daily allowances (mg): adults and children over 4: 10; children under 4: 5; infants: 3; pregnant and nursing women: 10.

Side effects and overdosage
Very large doses—more than 20 gm a day—can cause diarrhea and water retention.

Pectin

○○○

Use
Diarrhea control agent that works by adsorption. It is derived from citrus fruits or apples and is also used as an emulsifier in the food industry.

Where found
Kao-Paverin (with **kaolin** and bismuth subcarbonate).

Recommended dosage
Follow manufacturer's recommendations.

Side effects and overdosage
Well tolerated.

Permethrin

○○○

Use
Kills head and pubic lice. Sometimes used as an insect repellent on fabric. This is a synthetic form of **pyrethrins** and is also used in farming and veterinary medicine.

Where found
Nix cream rinse for lice. Also found in products such as Permanone designed for use on clothing or tents as a tick repellent.

Recommended dosage
For lice, shampoo thoroughly, rinse, and dry hair. Apply enough of the liquid to fully saturate the hair and scalp, especially behind the ears and nape of the neck. Leave it on for 10 minutes and rinse out with water. Avoid the eyes. Do not use in children younger than 2 months. May need to be repeated, but wait for a week or two.

Side effects and overdosage
May cause skin irritation: redness, itching, or swelling. May cause allergic reactions, especially in those with ragweed allergies, and may worsen asthma. There have been reports of super lice resistant to this ingredient. See Chapter 24 (Skin, Hair, and Nails) for advice on how to treat these cases with **petrolatum.**

Petrolatum

○ ○ ○

Use
Semi solid greasy compound widely used as an ointment base for cosmetics. By itself it can be used as a skin protectant and dry skin product (moisturizer or emollient), and although extremely effective for these purposes, it is messy and difficult to remove.

Where found
Vaseline 100% Pure Petroleum Jelly and many generic products. Also in numerous moisturizers, external creams, lotions, and ointments in combination with other products.

Recommended dosage
For use on dry skin: apply after bathing to moist skin as needed.

Side effects and overdosage
May worsen skin infections and cause acne. Skin irritation, although rare, may occur.

Synonym
Petroleum jelly, white soft paraffin.

Phenazopyridine

OOO

Use
Urinary analgesic. Relieves burning, pain, urgency, and frequency of urination in urinary tract infections. *Must be used in conjunction with specific treatment to combat the infection.*

Where found
Azo-Dine, Azo-Standard, Baridium, Prodium, Re-Azo, Uristat, UroFemme.

Recommended dosage
Adults and children over 12 years: 200mg 3 times a day after meals. Do not use for longer than 2 days.

Side effects and overdosage
Will turn urine orange or red and may stain undergarments. Contact lenses can also turn color. May cause upset stomach, headache, and skin rashes. Liver, kidney, and blood diseases may occur with large doses or in those with kidney failure.

Phenindamine

OOO

Use
Antihistamine (H_1 receptor) in the piperidine class.

Where found
Nolahist Tablets.

Recommended dosage
Adults and children over 12 years: 25 mg every 4 to 6 hours, not to exceed 150 mg per day. Children 6 to under 12 years: ½ the adult dose. Children 2 to under 6 years: ¼ the adult dose. Do not take the last dose after about 4 PM and avoid if you are pregnant or nursing.

Side effects and overdosage

Generally well tolerated but unlike most antihistamines phenindamine may cause stimulation even in adults. Some side effects, such as drowsiness, are undesirable when you are taking it during the day and want to stay awake, but desirable when you are taking it at night. Similarly, a dry nose may be uncomfortable unless you have a cold. Uncommon side effects include allergies, itching, rash, abnormal sensitivity to sunlight (photosensitivity), sweating, chills, nervousness, excitability (especially in children), blurred vision, upset stomach, nausea, vomiting, constipation, diarrhea, difficulty with urination, thickening of lung secretions, and wheezing. The sedative effect can be marked with alcohol, so avoid this combination. Older people are more sensitive to these side effects. Don't take any antihistamine if you have glaucoma, heart disease, thyroid disease, an enlarged prostate, diabetes, or high blood pressure. Check with your doctor if you have a lung disease such as asthma, emphysema, or chronic bronchitis. Also do not take antihistamines with other sleeping aids, tranquilizers, or antidepressants such as monoamine oxidase inhibitors (MAOIs).

Synonym
Phenindamine tartrate.

Pheniramine

ooo

Use
Antihistamine (H_1 receptor) in the alkylamine class.

Where found
Scot-Tussin Original (with **phenylephrine, sodium salicylate, and caffeine**). Also in the decongestant eye drops Naphcon A, OcuHist, and Opcon-A (with **naphazoline**).

Recommended dosage
Adults and children over 12 years: 12.5 to 25 mg every 4 to 6 hours, not to exceed 150 mg per day. Children 6 to under 12 years: ½ the adult dose. Children 2 to under 6 years: ¼

the adult dose. Avoid if you are pregnant or nursing. Follow manufacturer's recommendations for topical use in the eyes.

Side effects and overdosage
Generally well tolerated and less sedating than **diphenhydramine.** Some side effects, such as drowsiness, are undesirable when you are taking it during the day and want to stay awake, but desirable when you are taking it at night. Similarly, a dry nose may be uncomfortable unless you have a cold. Uncommon side effects include allergies, itching, rash, abnormal sensitivity to sunlight (photosensitivity), sweating, chills, nervousness, excitability (especially in children), blurred vision, upset stomach, nausea, vomiting, constipation, diarrhea, difficulty with urination, thickening of lung secretions, and wheezing. The sedative effect can be marked with **alcohol,** so avoid this combination. Older people are more sensitive to these side effects. Don't take any antihistamine if you have glaucoma, heart disease, thyroid disease, an enlarged prostate, diabetes, or high blood pressure. Check with your doctor before taking if you have a lung disease such as asthma, emphysema, or chronic bronchitis. Also do not take antihistamines with other sleeping aids, tranquilizers, or antidepressants such as monoamine oxidase inhibitors (MAOIs).

Synonym
Pheniramine maleate.

Phenol
○○○

Use
Phenol was the very first antiseptic to be used in surgery. Today it is employed in weak concentrations as a counterirritant, a local anesthetic, and antiseptic (preservative) in OTC preparations. In high concentrations it has been used by some plastic surgeons and dermatologists as a chemical peeling agent for facial wrinkles.

Where found
Numerous external analgesics, sore throat and sore mouth preparations, some insulins, some first aid products.

Recommended dosage
Follow manufacturer's recommendations. Do not cover a phenol containing compound with a bandage or other occlusive device.

Side effects and overdosage
Phenol is highly caustic, corrosive, and poisonous. Fatal liver and kidney disease has resulted from ingestion, prolonged skin contact, or inhalation of vapors. When used as directed in the available weak OTC products, however, it probably has few side effects, although there have been reports of severe breathing difficulties due to swelling of the throat in people who have used phenol containing throat sprays.

Synonym
Carbolic acid.

Phenylbenzimidazole sulfonic acid
○○○

Use
Sunscreen effective against UVB.

Where found
Several combination sunscreens.

Recommended dosage
Follow manufacturer's recommendations.

Side effects and overdosage
May cause skin irritation.

323

Phenylephrine

OOO

Use
Decongestant that works by narrowing blood vessels. Such drugs are called vasoconstrictors. Also has general stimulant effect on the nervous system that mimics **epinephrine**.

Where found
Among nasal decongestant sprays and drops Neo-Synephrine is the best known brand name that contains phenylephrine. It is also found in Dristan, Rhinall, Vicks Sinex Ultra Fine Mist, and others. In systemic cough and cold remedies it is in Cerose-DM, Codimal, Coldonyl, Dallergy-D, Dristan Cold Multi-Symptom, Emagrin Forte, Gendecon, Histatab Plus, ND-Gesic, Novahistine, Quelidrine, Scot-Tussin Original, and Spec-T Sore Throat Decongestant. In hemorrhoidal remedies it is present in Anusert, Hemorid, Hem-Prep, Medicone, and Preparation H. In eye decongestants it is in Ak-Nefrin, IsoptoFrin, Prefrin Liquifilm, Relief, and Zincfrin.

Recommended dosage
Orally: adults and children over 12 years: 10 mg every 4 hours as needed, not to exceed 60 mg per day; children 6 to under 12 years: ½ the adult dose; children 2 to under 6 years: ¼ the adult dose. For eye, nose, and hemorrhoidal products, follow manufacturer's directions. Avoid if you are pregnant or nursing. Avoid if you have heart disease, high blood pressure, thyroid disease, diabetes, or an enlarged prostate.

Side effects and overdosage
When taken orally it may cause nervousness, insomnia, palpitations, headache, dizziness, or irritability. Do not take with the antidepressants known as monoamine oxidase inhibitors (MAOIs) or for 2 weeks after stopping an MAOI. When used topically the main side effect is local irritation and rebound congestion, in which repeated use causes a widening of blood vessels and aggravation of symptoms.

Phenylpropanolamine

OOO

Use
Decongestant and appetite suppressant. As a decongestant, it works by narrowing blood vessels. Such drugs are called vasoconstrictors. Also has stimulant effects that mimic adrenaline (epinephrine) and is the only FDA approved drug for weight loss control. It is also a drug of abuse—in street lingo, a poor man's upper.

Where found
As a decongestant it is almost always combined with an antihistamine, analgesic, cough suppressant, or mucus liquefying agent such as in the following products and product lines: A.R.M., some Alka-Seltzer products, some BC products, Bromatapp Extended Release Tablets, Bromotap, Cheracol Plus, Comtrex (some), Contac (some), Coricidin D, Demazin, Dimetapp (many), Ipsatol, Kophane Cough and Cold Medicine, Naldecon (many), Pediacon DX, Prominocol, Propagest, Pyrroxate, Robitussin-CF, Sinapils, Sinulin, Tavist-D Antihistamine/Nasal Decongestant, Tri-Nefrin Extra Strength, Triaminic (some), Tricodene (some), and some Vicks products. As an appetite suppressant it is found in Acutrim, Amfed, Dexatrim, Dieutrim, Mini Slims, Mini-Thin, Permathene products, Protrim, Super Odrinex, Thinz Back-To-Nature, and Thinz-Span.

Recommended dosage
As a decongestant: adults and children over 12 years: 25 mg every 4 hours as needed, not to exceed 150 mg per day; children 6 to under 12 years: ½ the adult dose; children 2 to under 6 years: ¼ the adult dose. As an appetite suppressant: adults over 18 years: 75 mg timed release product per day. Do not take for longer than 3 months. Avoid if you are pregnant or nursing. Avoid with caffeine, ephedrine, phenylephrine, pseudoephedrine, and drugs taken for psychiatric problems such as the antidepressants known as monoamine oxidase inhibitors (MAOIs). Beta-blocker drugs such as propranolol (Inderal) or metoprolol (Lopressor) will increase the effects of this drug. Do not take if you have high

blood pressure, heart disease, thyroid disease, prostatic enlargement, or diabetes. Phenylpropanolamine will decrease the effects of the blood pressure medicines mecamylamine, methyldopa, and reserpine. As a general rule, do not take with any prescription drug unless directed by your doctor.

Side effects and overdosage
Generally well tolerated in recommended doses, but it may cause rapid or irregular heart rate, palpitations, insomnia, restlessness, headache, irritability, fear, anxiety, tenseness, tremor, weakness, pallor, difficulty breathing, painful or difficult urination. High doses may cause high blood pressure, stroke, heart attacks, and convulsions. Palpitations, in particular, may be an indication that your body cannot tolerate this drug or the dose of it you are taking.

Synonym
PPA.

Phenyltoloxamine

ooo

Use
Antihistamine (H_1 receptor) in the ethanolamine class. It is usually not listed as an active ingredient in the currently available products because it is designed to enhance the effects of internal analgesics. Phenyltoloxamine has conditional FDA approval because of insufficient data.

Where found
Percogesic (with **acetaminophen**) and Mobigesic (with **magesium salicylate**).

Recommended dosage
Follow manufacturer's recommendations.

Side effects and overdosage
Whether a given effect of an antihistamine is a side effect depends upon your reason for taking it. As a general rule it

is well tolerated. Some effects, such as drowsiness, are undesirable when you are taking it during the day and want to stay awake, but desirable when you are taking it to go to sleep. Similarly, a dry nose may be uncomfortable unless you have a cold. Many other side effects have been reported, however, including itching, rash, abnormal sensitivity to sunlight (photosensitivity), sweating, chills, nervousness, excitability (especially in children), blurred vision, upset stomach, nausea, vomiting, constipation, diarrhea, difficulty with urination, thickening of lung secretions, and wheezing. The sedative effect can be marked with **alcohol,** so avoid this combination. Older people are more sensitive to these side effects. Don't take any antihistamine if you have glaucoma, heart disease, thyroid disease, an enlarged prostate, diabetes, or high blood pressure. Check with your doctor before taking antihistamines if you have lung diseases such as asthma, emphysema, or chronic bronchitis. Also do not take antihistamines with other sleeping aids, tranquilizers, or antidepressants such as monoamine oxidase inhibitors (MAOIs).

Phosphorus

○ ○ ○

Use
Also known as phosphate (a salt form of phosphorus) this nutritional supplement is crucial to a wide variety of bodily functions and is a major component of bone, where it exists with calcium as calcium phosphate. Deficiency is very rarely a result of malnutrition because phosphorus is so widely available. Those taking large doses of **aluminum hydroxide,** however, may experience it, as might those with severe diabetes. Low phosphorus can lead to weakness, fatigue, and loss of appetite.

Where found
Grains, milk, eggs, meat, fish, nuts, seeds, and nutritional supplements.

Recommended dosage

Recommended daily allowances (mg): adults over 24 and children 1 to 10: 800; children and adults 11 to 24 and pregnant or nursing women: 1200.

Side effects and overdosage

Although toxicity from large doses is not recognized there is no reason to take phosphorus supplements unless your doctor directs you to do so.

Phosphorylated carbohydrate solution

OOO

Use

Control of nausea, vomiting, and upset stomach.

Where found

Cola, Emecheck, Emetrol, and Rakemetrol.

Recommended dosage

Adults and children over 12 years: 15 to 30 ml (1 to 2 tablespoons) every 15 minutes until vomiting stops. Do not take more than 5 doses per hour. If vomiting does not stop after 5 doses call your doctor.

Side effects and overdosage

Some of these products contain lots of sugar in the form of fructose, glucose, or sucrose. Care should be taken if you have diabetes.

Piperonyl butoxide

OOO

Use

Prevents lice from detoxifying **pyrethrins**.

Where found
See pyrethrins.

Recommended dosage
Follow manufacturer's recommendations.

Side effects and overdosage
May cause skin and eye irritation.

Poloxamer 407

OOO

Use
The poloxamers are chemicals that generally promote solubility and prevent foaming. The 407 type is used in dental cleansers and eye medications.

Where found
Orajel Baby Tooth & Gum Cleanser and some eye products.

Recommended dosage
Follow manufacturer's recommendations.

Side effects and overdosage
No reports of adverse effects.

Polyethylene glycol

OOO

Use
A series of chemicals that mainly function as solvents and bases (vehicles) for delivering medications externally and for increasing viscosity. Different numbers appended to the name (for example 200, 400, 1540, and 4000) represent different forms (molecular weights) of the substance with different qualities. The lower numbers, from 200 to 700, are

liquids, whereas the higher numbers, 1000 to 6000, are solids. These compounds are widely used in industry.

Where found
Numerous topical creams and liquids as well as eye drops. Also found in many shampoos, insect repellents, tooth-pastes, and suppositories.

Recommended dosage
Follow manufacturer's recommendations.

Side effects and overdosage
Generally well tolerated but some liquid forms (molecular weights from 200 to 400) may cause skin irritation.

Synonym
PEG.

Polymyxin B
ooo

Use
Antibiotic effective against some gram-negative bacteria.

Where found
Betadine First Aid Antibiotics Ointment, Campho-phenique Triple Antibiotic, Clomycin, Lanabiotic, Medi-Quik Triple Antibiotic, Mycitracin, Neosporin, Polysporin, Tri-Biozene, and Tribiotic Plus, all in combination with **bacitracin** or **neomycin** or both.

Recommended dosage
Apply 2 to 3 times a day.

Side effects and overdosage
Generally well tolerated.

Synonym
Polymyxin B sulfate.

Polyvinyl alcohol

O O O

Use
Vehicle and viscosity agent in eye products.

Where found
Several artificial tears and contact lens products.

Recommended dosage
Follow manufacturer's recommendations.

Side effects and overdosage
Well tolerated when used as directed.

Potassium nitrate

O O O

Use
Desensitizer for sensitive teeth that works by preventing transmission of cold, hot, pressure, or sweet sensations through the tooth.

Where found
Sensodyne is the best known product line, but potassium nitrate is also contained in a number of other toothpastes labelled for sensitive teeth. A 5 percent concentration is approved for OTC use; 10 percent concentrations are used in dentist's offices.

Recommended dosage
Apply a film to exposed surfaces with a soft toothbrush and leave on for 1 minute 2 times a day. May take up to 2 weeks to work. Do not use in children under 12 and do not use unless directed by a dentist. Do not swallow and do not use for long periods of time.

Side effects and overdosage
Well tolerated in recommended doses.

Synonym
Saltpeter.

Potassium salicylate

o o o

Use
Salicylate analgesic.

Where found
Diurex Long Acting (with **acetaminophen** and **caffeine**) and
Diurex Water Pills (with **salicylamide** and **caffeine**.)

Recommended dosage
Follow manufacturer's recommendations.

Side effects and overdosage
See **aspirin**.

Povidone

o o o

Use
Povidone refers to a group of synthetic compounds that
dissolve in water to produce a colloidal solution. They are
used as dispersing and suspending agents. In artificial tears
povidone is classified as a demulcent (something that coats
and protects mucous membranes).

Where found
Combined with **polyvinyl alcohol** and/or **cellulose ethers** in
several artificial tear liquid products.

Recommended dosage
For artificial tears: 1 or 2 drops in affected eyes as needed.

Side effects and overdosage
None reported.

Povidone-iodine

O O O

Use
Antiseptic effective against bacteria and fungi. The **povidone** holds and disburses the **iodine**.

Where found
The brand name Betadine is practically synonymous with this ingredient, and preparations are available as skin cleansers, topical applications, and vaginal douches. It is also present in the following douches: Massengill Medicated Disposable, Summer's Eve, Vaginex, and Yeast-Gard (some). In addition, the antifungals Aerodine, Minidyne, and Polydine contain it.

Recommended dosage
Follow manufacturer's recommendations.

Side effects and overdosage
Well tolerated when used as directed, but may cause skin and eye irritation.

Pramoxine

O O O

Use
Local anesthetic that is chemically unrelated to other types of local (-caine) anesthetics.

Where found
Hemorrhoidal products: Anusol Ointment, Fleet Pain-Relief, Hemorid for Women (cream & ointment, with **phenylephrine**), ProctoFoam, Tronothane. Skin (poison ivy, burn, and sunburn) products: Aveeno Anti-Itch, Anti-Itch, Caladryl, Dermatox, Itch-X, Pramegel, Prax, and others.

Recommended dosage
Adults and children over 12 years: Apply a 1 percent preparation every 4 hours as needed up to 5 times a day. Do not use for longer than 7 days.

Side effects and overdosage
Well tolerated when used as directed but may cause irritation of the mucous membranes or eyes.

Propylene glycol
○ ○ ○

Use
A very widely used solvent, vehicle, antiseptic, preservative, demulcent, and humectant. Also used as an emulsifier in foods and as a solvent for food colors.

Where found
Many topical preparations for the skin and mucous membranes, as well as some products taken internally.

Recommended dosage
Follow manufacturer's recommendations.

Side effects and overdosage
May cause irritation in some individuals externally, but tends to safe, even when taken internally.

Propylhexedrine

O O O

Use
Decongestant that works by narrowing blood vessels as a vasoconstrictor.

Where found
Benzedrex Nasal Inhaler (with **menthol**).

Recommended dosage
Adults and children over 12 years: 2 inhalations in each nostril every 2 hours as needed. Children 6 to under 12 years: ½ the adult dose with adult supervision. Do not use for longer than 7 days. Avoid if you are pregnant or nursing.

Side effects and overdosage
May cause burning, stinging, sneezing, increased nasal discharge, and irritation. Do not use if you have heart disease, high blood pressure, thyroid disease, diabetes, or an enlarged prostate. Rebound congestion, in which reflex dilatation of blood vessels causes persistant nasal stuffiness despite ever-increasing doses, may occur.

Pseudoephedrine

O O O

Use
Decongestant that works by narrowing blood vessels. Such drugs are called vasoconstrictors. Also has stimulant effects that mimic **epinephrine**.

Where found
The brand name Sudafed is practically synonymous with this product but it is found in many other allergy, cough and cold preparations, alone or in combination with antihistamines, analgesics, **dextromethorphan**, and **guaiafenesin**. The combination of pseudoephedrine and an antihistamine is

particularly common. Some of the products and product lines that contain it are: Actifed (most), Advil Cold & Sinus, Alka-Seltzer (many), Allerest products, Bayer Select Aspirin Free Sinus Relief, Benadryl products (many), Benylin Multi-Symptom Formula, Bromfed, Chlor-Trimeton (many), Codimal, Comtrex (many), Congestac, Contac (many), Creomulsion, DayGel, Dimacol, Dimetapp (many), Disophrol, Dorcol, Dristan (some), Drixoral (many), Dynafed, Efidac 24, Excedrin, Fedahist, Guaifed, GuiaCough PE, Guiatuss Cold & Cough, Hayfebrol, Kodet-SE, Kolephrin, Napril, Nasal D, NiteGel, Novahistine, Oranyl, Ornex, PediaCare products, Robitussin products (many), Sinarest products, Sine-Aid, Sine-Off, Singlet, Sinutab, Sinutol, Sudanyl, Tetrahist, TheraFlu, Tri-Fed, Triaminic (many), Tussar, Tylenol (many), and Vicks (many).

Recommended dosage
Adults and children over 12 years: 60 mg every 4 to 6 hours as needed, not to exceed 240 mg a day. Children 6 to under 12 years: ½ the adult dose. Children 2 to under 6 years: ¼ the adult dose. Timed release doses are available that deliver 120 mg over 12 hours or 240 mg over 24 hours (Efidac/24). Avoid if you are pregnant or nursing or if you have heart disease, high blood pressure, thyroid disease, diabetes, or an enlarged prostate. Do not take with the antidepressants known as monoamine oxidase inhibitors (MAOIs), such as Nardil (phenelzine), or for 2 weeks after stopping an MAOI.

Side effects and overdosage
May cause nervousness, excitability, insomnia, palpitations, headache, dizziness, or irritability.

Psyllium

OOO

Use
Bulk forming laxative. It usually works in 12 to 24 hours but may take as long as 3 days. Sometimes used under medical supervision to aid in lowering cholesterol.

Where found
By itself: Hydrocil Instant, Konsyl, Konsyl-D, Konsyl-Orange, Metamucil products (most), Modane Bulk, Perdiem Fiber, and Serutan. Also found in some products along with **senna** or **glycerin.**

Recommended dosage
Highly individualized. The adult dose range is 2.5 to 30 gm a day as needed, but follow manufacturer's directions for the recommended dose in a particular preparation and for use in children. Always take with at least 8 oz of water, fruit juice, soda, or other liquid. More liquid is even better. Do not use for longer than 1 week. Do not take if you have difficulty swallowing.

Side effects and overdosage
The most serious side effect is blockage of the esophagus (the tube that leads from the throat to the stomach) or choking if not enough fluid is taken. Many of these products also contain varying amounts of sodium and carbohydrate, which you should note if you are on a low sodium or weight loss diet or are diabetic. Psyllium may cause excess intestinal gas.

Synonyms
Plantago, plantain, ispaghula, psyllium hydrophilic mucilloid.

Pyrantel pamoate

○ ○ ○

Use
Kills pinworms *(Enterobius vermicularis)* by paralyzing the muscles the parasite uses to hold on to the walls of the intestine.

Where found
Antiminth, Pin-X, and Reese's Pinworm.

Recommended dosage

Adults and children 2 and over: 5 mg per pound (11 mg per kilogram) taken as a single dose, not to exceed 1 gm. For children under 2 or who weigh less than 25 pounds, check with your doctor. Similarly, if you have liver disease consult with a doctor first. Avoid if you are pregnant or nursing.

Side effects and overdosage

Generally well tolerated. Call your doctor if you develop nausea, vomiting, abdominal cramps, diarrhea, dizziness, or drowsiness.

Pyrethrins

ooo

Use

Insecticide derived from pyrethrum (chrysanthemum) flowers. Kills lice.

Where found

A-200, End-Lice, InnoGel Plus, Licetrol, Licide, Pronto, R&C, Rid, and Tegrin-LT Lice Killing Shampoo. In these products it is combined with **piperonyl butoxide.**

Recommended dosage

Apply to affected area and leave on for 10 minutes. Rinse out thoroughly with water. Repeat in 7 days. Avoid the eyes and other mucous membranes.

Side effects and overdosage

Usually well tolerated but may cause skin irritation: redness, itching, or swelling. May cause allergic reactions, especially in those with ragweed allergies, and may aggravate asthma. If taken internally can cause nausea, vomiting, ringing in the ears, and headaches. Some lice have developed a resistance to this chemical. See Chapter 24 (Skin, hair, and nails) for using **petrolatum** in such cases.

Synonyms

Pyrethroids, pyrethrum extract.

Pyrilamine

○○○

Use
Antihistamine (H_1 receptor) in the ethylenediamine class.

Where found
In Codimal, ND-Gesic, Robitussin Night Relief, Tricodene No. 1 combined with various decongestants, analgesics, and cough suppressants. It is also found in most Midol products and Diurex PMS along with **acetaminophen** and **pamabrom.**

Recommended dosage
Adults and children over 12 years: 25 to 50 mg every 6 to 8 hours, not to exceed 200 mg per day. Children 6 under 12 years: ½ the adult dose. Children 2 to under 6 years: ¼ the adult dose. Avoid if you are pregnant or nursing.

Side effects and overdosage
Pyrilamine tends to be somewhat less sedating than other antihistamines, but upset stomach may be more pronounced. Some side effects, such as drowsiness, are undesirable when you are taking it during the day and want to stay awake, but desirable when you are taking it at night. Similarly, a dry nose may be uncomfortable unless you have a cold. Uncommon side effects include allergies, itching, rash, abnormal sensitivity to sunlight (photosensitivity), sweating, chills, nervousness, excitability (especially in children), blurred vision, upset stomach, nausea, vomiting, constipation, diarrhea, difficulty with urination, thickening of lung secretions, and wheezing. The sedative effect can be marked with **alcohol,** so avoid this combination. Older people are more sensitive to these side effects. Don't take any antihistamine if you have glaucoma, heart disease, thyroid disease, an enlarged prostate, diabetes, or high blood pressure. If you have a lung disease such as asthma, emphysema, or chronic bronchitis, check with your doctor before taking antihistamines. Also do not take antihistamines with other sleeping aids, tranquilizers, or antidepressants such as monoamine oxidase inhibitors (MAOIs).

Synonym
Pyrilamine maleate.

Pyrithione zinc

OOO

Use
Dandruff, seborrhea, and psoriasis control. How it works is not exactly known, but it does slow the rate of growth of skin cells (cytostatic).

Where found
Brylcreem Anti-Dandruff, DHS Zinc, Head & Shoulders (most), Sebulon, X-Seb, Zincon, ZNP Bar, and generics.

Recommended dosage
For shampoos: lather with water, rub into scalp, and leave in place for 5 minutes. Repeat every other day for 6 weeks, then as needed. For other products, follow manufacturer's directions. Approved strength for shampoos is 0.3 to 2 percent and 0.1 to 0.25 percent for products that are to be left on the scalp or skin.

Side effects and overdosage
Well tolerated when used as recommended.

Synonym
Zinc pyrithionate.

Pyrophosphates

OOO

Use
Inhibits formation of tartar (calculus) by interfering with calcification of plaque.

Where found
In many tartar control toothpastes.

Recommended dosage
Follow manufacturer's recommendations.

Side effects and overdosage
Generally well tolerated but may decalcify tooth enamel if used in too high a dosage.

Synonyms
Tetrapotassium pyrophosphate, tetrasodium pyrophosphate.

Ranitidine
o o o

Use
A histamine receptor antagonist that reduces stomach acid by inhibiting its production. Used for prevention and relief of heartburn, indigestion, and sour stomach.

Where found
Zantac 75.

Recommended dosage
Adults and children over 12 years: 75 mg 2 times a day as needed. Do not exceed 150 mg a day or take for longer than 2 weeks. Avoid if you are pregnant or nursing. Prescription doses for more serious intestinal problems, such as ulcers, can range up to 300 mg a day.

Side effects and overdosage
Generally well tolerated but may cause headache, dizziness, nausea, and diarrhea. Larger doses, especially in the elderly, may cause mental disturbances, heart, liver, or blood problems.

Resorcinol

OOO

Use
A substance classified as a keratolytic that disrupts the bonds between skin cells and softens skin protein (keratin). The resulting damaged skin tends to slough off easily. This is sometimes helpful in allowing other ingredients to penetrate into the skin. Resorcinol is used for acne and itching.

Where found
Acne products: combined with **sulfur** in Acne Treatment Wash, Acne Treatment Tinted, Acnomel, Acnotex, Clearasil Adult Care, Rezamid, and Sulforcin. Anti-itch products: combined with **benzocaine** in Bicozene Creme External Analgesic and Vagisil. Also in Rid-Itch (with **benzoic acid** and **chlorothymol**) and Resinol Medicated Ointment (with **zinc oxide**).

Recommended dosage
Apply externally following manufacturer's directions.

Side effects and overdosage
May irritate skin, increase skin pigment, and darken hair. If applied to large or open areas may enter the bloodstream and cause toxic reactions, including convulsions. Green discoloration of the urine has been reported after applying large amounts.

Salicylamide

OOO

Use
Internal analgesic. This is an old compound of very questionable value that has been used for pain, fever, and inflammation. Although chemically related to **aspirin** it is not metabolized to **salicylic acid** in the same way.

Where found

Anodynos, BC powders, Emagrin, and Stanback (all with **aspirin** and **caffeine**). In Diurex Water Pills (with **potassium salicylate** and **caffeine**) and Fendol (with **phenylephrine, acetaminophen, guaiafenesin,** and **caffeine**.)

Recommended dosage

Follow manufacturer's recommendations for combination products. By itself, the recommended dosage is 325 to 650 mg 3 or 4 times a day for adults over the age of 15. These doses are less than those thought to be effective (1000 to 2000 mg every 4 hours).

Side effects and overdosage

None reported in OTC recommended doses.

Salicylic acid

OOO

Use

Softens skin by breaking down the protein keratin, which forms the bulk of the topmost layer of the skin. This effect is called keratolytic. Used in acne medications, dandruff and seborrhea control shampoos, psoriasis control preparations, and wart removers.

Where found

In low concentrations it is present in many acne preparations such as impregnated pads, liquids, and washes and in many dandruff shampoos. It is often combined with **sulfur** and sometimes with **coal tar**. In wart remover liquids it is generally in 17 percent concentration and in wart remover pads in a 40 percent concentration. It can also be found in some cosmetic wrinkle creams as a beta hydroxy acid.

Recommended dosage

Follow manufacturer's recommendations.

Side effects and overdosage

Irritates skin and causes peeling, the amount of which depending upon the strength and the amount applied.

Saline

ooo

Use

Irrigating solution for wounds and eyes. In concentrated form (2 percent and 5 percent) saline is used for chronic swelling of the cornea.

Where found

Widely available in generic and brand name forms.

Recommended dosage

Normal saline may be used liberally to cleanse or irrigate wounds or eye injuries. It should not be used as an eye drop over a prolonged period. Concentrated saline for swelling of the cornea should be used only under the direction of a doctor.

Side effects and overdosage

There are no side effects for the 0.9 percent solution, but concentrated preparations cause stinging. Homemade contact lens saline preparations from salt tablets may be hazardous because of contamination.

Synonym

Any solution of salt (sodium chloride) can be called saline, but the word saline usually refers to the 0.9 percent concentration, which is also called normal saline or physiologic saline, because it is roughly the same concentration of salt found in blood and other body fluids. The concentrated forms are called hypertonic saline. In homeopathic remedies salt is called natrium chloratum.

Selenium

○ ○ ○

Use

Nutritional supplement. Selenium is an element that is important to several enzyme systems in the body. Selenium deficiency may cause muscle weakness, including weakness of the heart (cardiomyopathy). Low selenium is usually found in those who have undergone prolonged intravenous feeding when selenium has not been added to the nutrient mixture. It is also found in geographic areas with low soil selenium. High selenium is associated with industrial exposure and in geographic areas with high soil selenium.

Where found

Seafood, grains, meat, dairy, and poultry products, and nutritional supplements.

Recommended dosage

Recommended daily allowance (mg): adults and children over 7: 0.05 to 0.2; children 4 to 6: 0.03 to 0.12; children 1 to 3: 0.02 to 0.08; infants 6 months to 1 year: 0.02 to 0.06; birth to 6 months: 0.01 to 0.04.

Side effects and overdosage

Selenium toxicity produces nervous system abnormalities, a garlic odor to the breath, and swelling of the hands and feet.

Selenium sulfide

○ ○ ○

Use

Dandruff, seborrhea, and psoriasis control. How it works is not exactly known, but it is generally thought to reduce the rate at which cells divide (cytostatic). Also has some antifungal activity, and in concentrated forms (2.5 percent) it can be used to treat the common sun fungus called tinea versicolor.

Where found
Head & Shoulders Intensive Treatment and Selsun Blue in 1 percent strengths. 2.5 percent preparations are available by prescription.

Recommended dosage
Wet hair and lather well, leaving it in contact with the scalp for 3 to 5 minutes. This may be preceeded by a normal shampooing. Use every other day for 6 weeks and as needed thereafter.

Side effects and overdosage
Generally well tolerated but can be toxic if taken internally. May irritate the skin and particularly the eyes. May discolor hair and make it more oily. Although there are reports of hair loss from using selenium sulfide shampoos, this probably does not occur.

Senna
ooo

Use
Stimulant type laxative usually effective in 6 to 12 hours. This is an old remedy in the anthraquinone class of laxatives.

Where found
Alone in Correctol Herbal Tea, Dr. Caldwell Senna, Ex-Lax, Fletcher's Castoria, Senokot, Senolax, and generics. With **psyllium** in Garfield's Tea and Innerclean Herbal, Perdiem, and Swiss Kriss. Also may be found combined with the stool softener **docusate**.

Recommended dosage
Follow manufacturer's recommendations and use the smallest amount possible. Available in a variety of tablets, syrups, granules, teas, and suppositories. Do not use for longer than 1 week. Avoid if you are pregnant or nursing.

Side effects and overdosage
May discolor the colon and the urine.

Synonyms
Senna concentrate, sennosides A & B.

Shark liver oil

○○○

Use
Protectant in hemorrhoidal preparations.

Where found
Preparation H products, Prompt Relief, and Wyanoids Relief Factor.

Recommended dosage
Follow manufacturer's recommendations.

Side effects and overdosage
Well tolerated.

Silica

○○○

Use
Dentifrice abrasive.

Where found
Many toothpastes, tooth gels, and tooth powders.

Recommended dosage
Brush 2 times a day for 2 minutes.

Side effects and overdosage
Excessively vigorous brushing can damage the softer parts of teeth if they are exposed.

Synonym
Silicon dioxide.

Silicone

○ ○ ○

Use
Skin protectant that tends to stick well to skin while repelling water.

Where found
Various diaper rash and dry skin products.

Recommended dosage
Follow manufacturer's recommendations.

Side effects and overdosage
Safe but may irritate raw, abraded, or traumatized skin.

Synonym
Dimethicone.

Simethicone

○ ○ ○

Use
The only FDA approved remedy for excessive gas. It works as a defoaming agent by reducing the surface tension of gas bubbles in the stomach and intestines, allowing them to break apart or come together to be expelled more easily. Opinion is divided as to its effectiveness.

Where found
By itself in Alka-Seltzer Anti-Gas, Gas-X, Maalox Anti-Gas, Mylanta Gas Relief, Phazyme Gas Relief, and generics. In combination with many antacids, usually signified by an additional word: plus or anti-gas. Pediatric preparations are available, such as Little Tummys Infant Gas Relief and Infant's Mylicon.

Recommended dosage
Adults and children over 12 years: 80 to 250 mg after meals and at bedtime as needed. Do not take more than 500 mg per day. Follow manufacturer's guidelines for pediatric dosing.

Side effects and overdosage
No known side effects.

Sodium bicarbonate
○○○

Use
Antacid and toothpaste abrasive. As an antacid, it reacts in the stomach with hydrochloric acid to form sodium chloride (salt) and carbon dioxide gas. When used in dentifrice products it tends to raise the pH (reducing the acidity) in the mouth. This is considered beneficial to the oral tissues.

Where found
Arm & Hammer Baking Soda and generic products, several antacids (see Chapter 16), and many toothpastes.

Recommended dosage
Follow manufacturer's recommendations. Avoid in pregnancy because of excess sodium.

Side effects and overdosage
Large amounts may cause fluid retention, which may include swelling of the legs, increase in blood pressure, and frequent urination. Also may reduce acidity in the blood (metabolic alkalosis) which may produce headache, loss of appetite, mental changes, and slow breathing. Excess stomach and intestinal gas is common.

Synonym
Baking soda.

Sodium borate

OOO

Use
Antiseptic, astringent, alkalinizer, and preservative.

Where found
Various eye drops and contact lens solutions.

Recommended dosage
Follow manufacturer's recommendations.

Side effects and overdosage
Generally well tolerated.

Synonym
Borax.

Sodium citrate

OOO

Use
Mucus liquefying agent (expectorant) and buffer in eye products (used to adjust the acidity).

Where found
Scot-Tussin Original and REM Liquid. Also in many eye preparations.

Recommended dosage
Follow manufacturer's recommendations.

Side effects and overdosage
Generally well tolerated.

Sodium diacetate

OOO

Use
Antiseptic.

Where found
Buro-Sol (with **benzethonium chloride**).

Recommended dosage
Follow manufacturer's recommendations.

Side effects and overdosage
Generally well tolerated.

Sodium edetate

OOO

Use
Antiseptic and preservative. Works by breaking down cell membranes, thus allowing other antiseptics to work.

Where found
As a preservative in some artificial tears, eye drops, and contact lens products.

Recommended dosage
Follow manufacturer's recommendations.

Side effects and overdosage
Generally well tolerated in the small amounts used.

Synonym
EDTA, disodium edetate.

Sodium fluoride

OOO

Use
Anti-cavity agent in dental products.

Where found
Present in numerous toothpastes, tooth gels, and tooth powders. Also present in topical fluoride products such as Fluorigard Anti-Cavity, Oral-B Anti-Cavity, and the Reach Act product line.

Recommended dosage
Follow manufacturer's guidelines. In powder form there may be insufficient fluoride delivered to the tooth surface. The liquid rinses should be swished in the mouth for one minute after brushing and spat out. Try not to eat or drink anything for 30 minutes afterward.

Side effects and overdosage
Excess fluoride may discolor and mottle teeth.

Sodium hypochlorite

OOO

Use
Antiseptic. Ordinary household bleach (such as Clorox) is a 5.25 percent sodium hypochlorite solution. OTC products designed for the skin should be no stronger than 0.5 percent.

Where found
Dakin's Solution.

Recommended dosage
Follow manufacturer's recommendations.

Side effects and overdosage
May irritate skin.

Sodium lauryl sulfate

OOO

Use
Surface active agent (detergent) that disburses ingredients and promotes foam and suds.

Where found
Present in many toothpastes, shampoos, vaginal lubricants, and douches.

Recommended dosage
Follow manufacturer's recommendations.

Side effects and overdosage
Well tolerated.

Sodium monofluorophosphate

OOO

Use
Anti-cavity agent in dental products.

Where found
Present in numerous toothpastes.

Recommended dosage
Brush teeth for 2 minutes 2 times a day. In powder form may not be delivered adequately to the tooth surface. Follow manufacturer's recommendations with regard to the extra-strength products, since they are not designed for children under 2. Should not be swallowed, and children under 6 years should be supervised while brushing teeth.

Side effects and overdosage
Excess fluoride may discolor and mottle teeth.

Sodium phosphate

○○○

Use
Saline type laxative. Works by drawing water into the intestine, increasing volume, and stimulating evacuation. Works in 30 minutes to 3 hours. Used for rapid emptying of the bowel before certain medical tests.

Where found
Fleet Ready-to-use-Enema and Phospho-soda Buffered Saline.

Recommended dosage
Follow manufacturer's recommendations for both oral and enema forms. Products are designed for single, one-time use. Avoid if you are pregnant or nursing.

Side effects and overdosage
Significant amounts of sodium may be absorbed through either the oral or rectal route and so these products should be used with caution if you are are on a sodium restricted diet.

Synonyms
Dibasic sodium phosphate, monobasic sodium phosphate.

Sodium salicylate

○○○

Use
Reduces pain, fever, and inflammation. Similar to, but less effective than, **aspirin.**

Where found
Cystex tablets (with **methenamine** and **benzoic acid**). Also in Scot-Tussin Original (with **phenylephrine, pheniramine,** and **caffeine**).

Recommended dosage
Adults and children over 15 years: 325 to 650 mg every 4 hours as needed, not to exceed 4000 mg a day. Do not take for longer than 10 days for pain or 3 days for fever. Avoid if you are on a sodium restricted diet. Do not give to children or teenagers with the symptoms of flu or chickenpox. Avoid in pregnancy, particularly in the last 3 months.

Side effects and overdosage
In general these are similar to **aspirin** except that this drug produces fewer allergic reactions and much less blood thinning.

Sorbic acid
○ ○ ○

Use
Antiseptic and preservative.

Where found
Replens (vaginal moisturizer) and many artificial tears and contact lens products.

Recommended dosage
Follow manufacturer's recommendations.

Side effects and overdosage
Generally well tolerated in the small amounts present in most products.

Sorbitol
○ ○ ○

Use
A form of sugar used as an artificial sweetener and as a moisturizer (humectant). Sometimes employed as a laxative

in high concentrations (up to 70 percent). Used in dentifrices because it does not promote cavities, but it does contain calories.

Where found
Several toothpastes, mouthwashes, and moisturizers.

Recommended dosage
Follow manufacturer's recommendations.

Side effects and overdosage
Generally well tolerated, but may cause diarrhea if ingested in very large amounts.

Stannous fluoride

O O O

Use
Anti-cavity agent in dental products.

Where found
Present in many toothpastes. In a stabilized form in Crest Gum Control.

Recommended dosage
Brush teeth for 2 minutes 2 times a day. In powder form insufficient fluoride may be delivered to the tooth surface, so pastes and gels are preferred.

Side effects and overdosage
Excess fluoride may discolor and mottle teeth.

Strontium chloride

O O O

Use
Tooth desensitizer.

Where found
Original Formula Sensodyne-SC, Thermodent.

Recommended dosage
Follow manufacturer's recommendations.

Side effects and overdosage
Generally well tolerated.

Sulfur

OOO

Use
Sulfur is an ancient drug that is generally classified as an antiseptic and keratolytic (something that softens the skin protein keratin). It is now used mostly OTC for acne and dandruff treatment.

Where found
By itself for acne: Acne Treatment Vanishing, Fostril, Liquimat, SAStid soap, Seales Lotion-Modified, Sulmasque, Sulpho-Lac, Sulray, and Thylox Acne Treatment Soap. Also found in a number of products combined with **resorcinol** or **salicylic acid**. By itself for dandruff and seborrhea: Sulfoam Medicated Antidandruff and Sulray products. Also found combined with **salicylic acid** and **coal tar** in a number of shampoos.

Recommended dosage
For acne: Apply 1 to 2 times a day. Do not spot treat. For dandruff and seborrhea: follow manufacturer's recommendations.

Side effects and overdosage
Usually well tolerated but may cause skin irritation. May also actually worsen acne, causing blackheads and whiteheads, if used over a prolonged period.

Synonym
Sulphur.

Talc

○○○

Use
Powder base used to absorb moisture and provide lubrication.

Where found
Many commercial powders.

Recommended dosage
Follow manufacturer's recommendations. Avoid inhaling particles.

Side effects and overdosage
Inhaling talc may lead to lung disease.

Synonym
Magnesium silicate.

Tetrachlorosalicylanilide

○○○

Use
Antiseptic.

Where found
Impregnon Concentrate.

Recommended dosage
This product is mainly designed to disinfect diapers. For cloth diapers dilute 5 ml (1 teaspoon) in a gallon of water and soak them before laundering. Although the manufacturer provides instructions for spraying on disposable diapers, this use cannot be recommended because of the potential for irritation.

Side effects and overdosage
May cause skin irritation if used on disposable diapers.

Tetrahydrozoline

OOO

Use
Decongestant that works by narrowing blood vessels as a vasoconstrictor.

Where found
In the following eye drops: Collyrium Fresh, Eye-Sed, EyeSine, Murine Plus, Optigene, Soothe, Visine (most), and generics.

Recommended dosage
Adults over 12 years: 1 to 2 drops in affected eye(s) up to 4 times a day. Do not use for longer than 3 days. If you have glaucoma check with your doctor. Avoid if you are pregnant or nursing.

Side effects and overdosage
May produce eye pain, blurry vision, or eye irritation and may sting when first applied. Rebound congestion, in which reflex widening (dilatation) of blood vessels causes persistent redness, may also occur.

Thimerosal

OOO

Use
Antiseptic and preservative, relatively weak.

Where found
In a few OTC nasal decongestants, artificial tears, contact lens products, and first aid preparations, but use is decreasing because of toxicity.

Recommended dosage
Follow manufacturer's recommendations.

Side effects and overdosage
Poisoning has occurred from applying thimerosal externally on open wounds. Severe allergic reactions can occur.

Thymol

OOO

Use
Antiseptic and preservative similar to **phenol**. Derived from the herb thyme and has an aroma that most people find pleasant.

Where found
Various aromatic products such as Vicks Vapo Rub, Listerine, and Massengil Unscented Vaginal Douche. Usually combined with other ingredients, such as **alcohol, eucalyptol, menthol, camphor, methyl salicylate,** and **turpentine.**

Recommended dosage
Follow manufacturer's recommendations.

Side effects and overdosage
Generally well tolerated in the weak concentrations found in most OTC preparations but by itself it is quite toxic, caustic, and poisonous, and may irritate skin and mucous membranes.

Synonym
Oil of thyme.

Tioconazole

OOO

Use
Single dose antifungal for vaginal yeast infections.

Where found
Vagistat-1

Recommended dosage
Insert one applicator-full into the vagina before bedtime.

Side effects and overdosage
Well tolerated but may cause vaginal burning and itching.

Titanium dioxide

○○○

Use
Sunblock with a broad range in both UVB and UVA bands. It is usually added to sunscreens to extend the spectrum of activity to include UVA. Also used in some toothpastes as a pigment to whiten teeth.

Where found
Neutrogena Chemical-Free Sunblocker, Presun 21, TI Screen, and many combination sunscreens.

Recommended dosage
Follow manufacturer's recommendations.

Side effects and overdosage
Well tolerated. There is evidence that the microfine form of titanium dioxide present in sunscreens is absorbed into the skin, but the effects of this absorption are not known.

Tolnaftate

○○○

Use
Antifungal for ringworm, jock itch, and athlete's foot. Not designed for ringworm of the scalp.

Where found
Aftate, Blis-To-Sol liquid, Fungicure gel, some Desenex and Absorbine jr. products, NP-27, Tinactin, Ting, Odor-Eaters, and Dr. Scholl's athlete's foot products.

Recommended dosage
Apply 2 times a day. Avoid the eyes.

Side effects and overdosage
Skin irritation is possible.

Triclosan
○○○

Use
Antiseptic. It is effective against gram positive bacteria (such as *Staphylococcus* and *Streptococcus)* and most gram negative bacteria, but weak against *Pseudomonas.*

Where found
Dial, Lever 2000, and other soaps and skin-care products labelled as having antibacterial qualities. Also in Total toothpaste.

Recommended dosage
Follow manufacturer's recommendations.

Side effects and overdosage
May produce skin irritation.

Tripelennamine
○○○

Use
Antihistamine in the ethylenediamine class. It is one of the oldest antihistamines but is only available OTC in external preparations. A prescription is needed for oral forms.

Where found
Di-Delamine gel and spray (with **diphenhydramine, menthol,** and **benzalkonium chloride).**

Recommended dosage
Follow manufacturer's recommendations.

Side effects and overdosage
May cause skin irritation.

Triprolidine

ooo

Use
Antihistamine (H_1 receptor) in the alkylamine class.

Where found
Some Actifed products, Cenafed Plus, Genac, and Tri-Fed, combined with **pseudoephedrine** and/or **acetaminophen.**

Recommended dosage
Adults and children over 12 years: 2.5 mg every 4 to 6 hours, not to exceed 10 mg per day. Children 6 to under 12 years: ½ the adult dose. Although triprolidine is the only OTC antihistamine approved for use in children under 2 years of age, it is best to check with your doctor before giving one of the available products to anyone under the age of 6. Avoid if you are pregnant or nursing.

Side effects and overdosage
Generally well tolerated. Some side effects, such as drowsiness, are undesirable when you are taking it during the day and want to stay awake, but desirable when you are taking it at night. Similarly, a dry nose may be uncomfortable unless you have a cold. Uncommon side effects include allergies, itching, rash, abnormal sensitivity to sunlight (photosensitivity), sweating, chills, nervousness, excitability (especially in children), blurred vision, upset stomach, nausea, vomiting, constipation, diarrhea, difficulty with urination, thick-

ening of lung secretions, and wheezing. The sedative effect can be marked with alcohol, so avoid this combination. Older people are more sensitive to these side effects. Don't take any antihistamine if you have glaucoma, heart disease, thyroid disease, an enlarged prostate, diabetes, or high blood pressure. Consult your doctor for use in lung diseases such as asthma, emphysema, or chronic bronchitis. Also do not take antihistamines with other sleeping aids, tranquilizers, or antidepressants such as monoamine oxidase inhibitors (MAOIs).

Synonym
Triprolidine hydrochloride.

Trolamine salicylate
○ ○ ○

Use
External analgesic that works by increasing salicylate levels in the tissues. It also has sunscreen properties in the UVB range.

Where found
Aspercreme, Mobisyl, Myoflex, and Sportscreme External Analgesic Rub. No sunscreens are currently available.

Recommended dosage
Adults over 15 years: apply 1 to 4 times a day as needed. Do not use for longer than 7 days; do not use if symptoms disappear and then reappear in a few days. Do not use in children or teenagers with symptoms of flu or chickenpox. Avoid if you are pregnant or nursing.

Side effects and overdosage
May cause skin irritation or other allergic reactions. Considerable absorption of salicylate may occur (see aspirin).

Turpentine

○○○

Use
Counterirritant in external analgesics obtained from pine tree resins. Medicinal turpentine is much purer than commercial turpentine and they are *not* interchangeable.

Where found
Sloan's Liniment (with **capsaicin**), Vick's VapoRub (with **camphor** and **menthol**, but the turpentine is considered inactive).

Recommended dosage
Adults and children over 2 years: apply 3 to 4 times a day as needed. Do not use for longer than 7 days.

Side effects and overdosage
Usually well tolerated when used as directed in the commercially available strengths, but some individuals are very allergic to it and develop severe skin irritation (contact dermatitis) with skin blistering. In higher concentrations or when used over large areas it can cause intestinal and breathing problems. Death has resulted from oral ingestion.

Synonyms
Turpentine oil, spirits of turpentine.

Undecylenate

○○○

Use
Antifungal for ringworm, jock itch, and athlete's foot. Not designed for scalp ringworm.

Where found
Blis-To-Sol powder, Cruex (some), Desenex (some), Fungi-Cure, Undelenic, generics.

Recommended dosage
Adults and children 2 years and older: apply 2 times a day, keeping away from the eyes. Discontinue if irritation develops.

Side effects and overdosage
Skin irritation—redness, burning, stinging, or scaling—is fairly common.

Synonym
Calcium undecylenate, undecylenic acid, zinc undecylenate.

Urea
○○○

Use
Keratolytic (something that disrupts the attachments between skin cells and softens skin protein). Allows penetration of other ingredients into the skin and aids moisturization.

Where found
Ultra Mide 25 Moisturizer contains the highest concentration—25 percent. Others are Carmol 10, Carmol 20, Eucerin Plus Creme, Gormel, Neutraplus, and Shepard's Skin Cream. Also found combined with other skin softeners such as **lactic acid.**

Recommended dosage
Follow manufacturer's recommendations.

Side effects and overdosage
May sting, especially if skin is irritated.

Vitamin A

OOO

Use

Vitamin A is a fat-soluble vitamin essential to the proper functioning of many organs, including the skin, immune system, and eyes. Vitamin A is not actually one chemical but a group of substances that have similar effects on the body and that have vitamin A activity. The main sources of vitamin A activity are the carotenoids, which include beta-carotene. Symptoms of low vitamin A include dryness of the eyes and decreased vision in low light. Severe vitamin A deficiency causes blindness and is, in fact, the main cause of blindness in the world. Low vitamin A is found with inadequate dietary intake or, more commonly in the U.S., intestinal malabsorption (in which the intestines fail to absorb nutrients properly). Vitamin A isn't actually needed every day because the liver stores a substantial supply of it.

Where found

Fish, dairy products, pigmented and green leafy vegetables, and nutritional supplements.

Recommended dosage

Recommended daily allowances (International Units): adults and children over 4: 5,000; children under 4: 2,500; infants: 1,500; pregnant and nursing women: 8,000.

Side effects and overdosage

High and potentially toxic doses of vitamin A have been used for many years by doctors to treat certain rare skin diseases. One related compound, called isotretinoin (Accutane), the most powerful and effective drug to treat acne, produces many of the same symptoms as high doses of vitamin A itself. But before you decide to take mega amounts to clear your complexion, be aware that by the time you note beneficial effects, you would have become extremely ill. Symptoms of toxicity include headache, dizziness, nausea, vomiting, dry skin, liver enlargement, joint pain, hair loss, fatigue, depression, and visual disturbances, such as double vision. Most dangerous for pregnant women, because high doses are associated with birth defects. Infants given large amounts can develop hydrocephalus (increased fluid pressure inside the brain). It should be noted that vitamin A toxicity is not the same as carotenemia, an orange hue to the skin seen in people who eat lots of carrots or pumpkins. Carotenemia is benign and not associated with other symptoms of vitamin A toxicity. A similar condition (lycopenemia) occurs from eating lots of tomatoes.

Vitamin B₁

ooo

Use
Vitamin B₁ is a water-soluble vitamin important to general metabolism, especially carbohydrate metabolism. There are many symptoms associated with deficiency, the classic disorder being called beriberi, in which nerve and heart disease are prominent. Low levels of vitamin B₁ can result from malnutrition, alcoholism, liver disease, and chronic diarrhea. Alcoholics, in particular, are notoriously prone to this deficiency.

Where found
Rice grain hulls, beans, peas, beef, pork, and nutritional supplements.

Recommended dosage
Recommended daily allowances (mg): adults and children over 4: 1.5; children under 4: 0.7; infants: 0.5; pregnant and nursing women: 1.7.

Side effects and overdosage
The only indications for high doses of vitamin B₁ are in certain rare hereditary enzyme deficiencies and in malnutrition. There is some evidence that larger doses than normal may relieve morning sickness in pregnancy, but check with your doctor before using it on your own.

Synonym
Thiamine.

Vitamin B$_{12}$

OOO

Use

Vitamin B$_{12}$ activity is present in a number of chemical compounds and is central to a wide variety of biological processes. It is present and active in all cells of the body. Symptoms of deficiency include weakness, numbness, tingling of the extremities, and loss of certain sensations. Poor nutrition—except in strict vegetarians—is rarely a cause of deficiency since this vitamin is so widely distributed in nature. Rather, the problem is usually poor absorption. Strict vegetarians should take supplemental vitamin B$_{12}$. Vitamin B$_{12}$ injections given by doctors should only be used to treat the condition known as pernicious anemia.

Where found

Meats, fish, milk, eggs, soy sauce, and nutritional supplements.

Recommended dosage

Recommended daily allowances (mcg): adults and children over 4: 6; children under 4: 3; infants: 2; pregnant and nursing women: 8.

Side effects and overdosage

Vitamin B$_{12}$ tends to be very safe even in high doses.

Synonym

Cyanocobalamin.

Vitamin B$_2$

OOO

Use

Vitamin B$_2$ is important to many body functions and is essential for growth. Symptoms of deficiency include inflammation of the mouth, tongue, throat, skin, and eyes, but often there are other problems related to deficiencies of the other B vitamins. Low vitamin B_2 may be seen with malnutrition and intestinal malabsorption, in which the intestines fail to absorb nutrients properly.

Where found
Meats, fish, dairy products, grains, dark green vegetables, and nutritional supplements.

Recommended dosage
Recommended daily allowances (mg): adults and children over 4: 1.7; children under 4: 0.8; infants: 0.6; pregnant and nursing women: 2.

Side effects and overdosage
May cause a yellow-orange discoloration of the urine in high doses.

Synonym
Riboflavin.

Vitamin B_6
○○○

Use
Vitamin B_6 is important to the immune system, nervous system, blood, and general metabolism. In infants, deficiency can cause irritability and seizures, particularly if formula has been heated excessively. In adults there can be confusion, numbness or tingling of the extremities, anemia, and skin rashes, but because there is usually a mixed deficiency with other B vitamins it can be hard to distinguish the symptoms of one vitamin B deficiency from another. Vitamin B_6 deficiency occurs in malnutrition, malabsorption (in which the intestines fail to absorb nutrients properly), pregnancy, alcoholism, and certain genetic diseases. Some prescription drugs, including birth control pills, may reduce vitamin B_6.

Where found

Meats, fish, grains, beans, peas, nuts, bananas, avocados, potatoes, green leafy vegetables, and nutritional supplements.

Recommended dosage

Recommended daily allowances (mg): adults and children over 4: 2; children under 4: 0.7; infants: 0.4; pregnant and nursing women: 2.5.

Side effects and overdosage

Vitamin B_6 toxicity may cause numbness, tingling, and clumsiness. High doses also inhibit the hormone prolactin, a subtance that stimulates women's breasts and men's reproductive organs. One may also become dependent upon such doses, leading to symptoms of deficiency upon withdrawal. Too much vitamin B_6 may affect the action of certain prescription drugs such as phenobarbital, phenytoin, and levodopa.

Synonyms

Pyridoxine, pyridoxal, pyridoxamine.

Vitamin C

O O O

Use

Vitamin C is important in the manufacture of collagen, one of the main structural components of the body. The classic deficiency state is called scurvy, the symptoms of which are fatigue, muscle aches, bleeding gums, bleeding into the skin, and poor wound healing. Deficiency states can occur in malnutrition, intestinal malabsorption, alcoholism, pregnancy, hyperthyroidism, and kidney disease. There is little evidence that vitamin C is good for the common cold.

Where found
Citrus fruits such as oranges, grapefruit, lemons, and limes, dark green vegetables, broccoli, tomatoes, potatoes, strawberries, melons, and nutritional supplements.

Recommended dosage
Recommended daily allowances (mg): adults and children over 4: 60; children under 4: 40; infants: 35; pregnant and nursing women: 60.

Side effects and overdosage
The body is able to metabolize only about 200 mg of vitamin C a day; the rest is excreted. There is no value, then, in doses higher than this, and most Americans who take multivitamins are close to the saturation point. High doses can cause kidney stones and anemia and may interfere with urine tests for sugar and with the action and excretion of other drugs, including antidepressants and anticoagulants (blood thinners). There have been reports of scurvy occurring in infants whose mothers took huge amounts of vitamin C while pregnant.

Synonym
Ascorbic acid.

Vitamin D

OOO

Use
Vitamin D is a fat-soluble vitamin that has many important functions, particularly in calcium and bone metabolism. There are a number of chemicals with vitamin D activity. The classic deficiency disease in children is called rickets, in which the bones soften and the joints become deformed. In adults, vitamin D deficiency may produce thinning of the bones, but both problems are very rare in the U. S. Certain medical problems, however, such as liver disease, kidney disease, or intestinal diseases, may cause decreased absorption of this vitamin.

Where found
Vitamin D is manufactured in the skin if enough sunlight is present. Milk, other dairy products, fish, and beef are other sources of the vitamin.

Recommended dosage
Recommended daily allowance (International Units): 400.

Side effects and overdosage
High doses of vitamin D may cause calcium imbalance, with increased levels of blood calcium and possibly kidney stones. Weakness, loss of appetite, weight loss, excessive urination, constipation, aches, pains, joint stiffness, and nausea are possible symptoms.

Vitamin E

000

Use
Vitamin E is a fat-soluble vitamin that is important to the nervous system. There are a number of chemical compounds that have vitamin E activity, the most active being alpha tocopherol. Deficiency is very rare. When it occurs it is seen mostly in children, either in very premature infants or in those with cystic fibrosis. Adults with intestinal malabsorption or intestinal bypass surgery may also have vitamin E deficiency, the main symptom of which is difficulty in sensing one's body position. Deficiency of this vitamin is almost never due to inadequate intake because it is so plentiful in nature, but rather as a result of poor intestinal absorption. If you are otherwise healthy, there is no reason to take supplements. Isolated studies have suggested that extra amounts might benefit the cardiovascular and immune systems, but these findings have not been confirmed.

Where found
Vegetable oils, green vegetables, nuts, grains, and nutritional supplements.

Recommended dosage

Recommended daily allowances (International Units): adults, children over 4: 30; children under 4: 10; infants: 5.

Side effects and overdosage

Those taking oral anticoagulants should not ingest supplemental vitamin E unless directed by a doctor.

Synonym

Tocopherol.

Vitamin K

○ ○ ○

Use

The term vitamin K refers to a group of chemical compounds that are important to the blood-clotting system. The symptom of deficiency is excessive bleeding, but it is very uncommon except in those who have debilitating diseases or who are otherwise very ill.

Where found

Liver, green leafy vegetables, cabbage, cauliflower, peas, potatoes, grains, and nutritional supplements. Vitamin K is also manufactured in the intestines by intestinal bacteria.

Recommended dosage

Recommended daily allowances (mcg): adults and children over 4: 20 to 80; children under 4: 15; infants: 5 to 10; pregnant and nursing women: 65.

Side effects and overdosage

Except in newborns, high doses of vitamin K appear to be safe. Those taking oral anticoagulants should not ingest supplemental vitamin K unless directed by a doctor.

Witch hazel

○○○

Use
Astringent. An old remedy derived from the twigs and leaves of *Hamamelis virginiana*, a shrub found in the eastern U.S. Most preparations have added **alcohol**, but some (mostly found in Europe), rely upon the tannic acid found naturally in the plant for the astringent effect.

Where found
Dickinson's Witch Hazel Compound and many hemorrhoidal products.

Recommended dosage
Apply as needed to weeping, oozing, or irritated skin.

Side effects and overdosage
Generally well tolerated but the alcohol may cause dryness or irritation.

Synonym
Hamamelis water.

Xylometazoline

○○○

Use
Nasal decongestant of medium (6 to 10 hours) duration. Works by narrowing blood vessels as a vasoconstrictor.

Where found
Otrivin (0.1 percent) and Otrivin Pediatric (0.05 percent).

Recommended dosage
0.1 percent solution: adults and children over 12 years: 2 to 3 drops or sprays every 8 to 10 hours. 0.05 percent solution:

adults and children over 2: 2 to 3 drops or sprays every 8 to 10 hours. Do not use for longer than 3 days. Avoid if you are pregnant or nursing. Do not use if you have heart disease, high blood pressure, thyroid disease, diabetes, or an enlarged prostate.

Side effects and overdosage
May cause burning, stinging, sneezing, increased nasal discharge, and irritation. Rebound congestion, in which reflex dilatation of blood vessels causes persistant nasal stuffiness despite ever-increasing doses, may occur but is less common than with shorter acting decongestants.

Zinc

OOO

Use
Normally present in the body in small amounts, zinc is crucial to numerous bodily functions. Zinc deficiency is characterized by poor wound healing, retarded growth, and atrophy of the reproductive organs. Zinc deficiency can be found in premature infants, malnutrition, in those whose intestines absorb zinc poorly (as in the disease called acrodermatitis enteropathica), or those in whom there is increased excretion (as in liver disease, kidney disease, or diabetes). Low zinc can also be present in AIDS and after heart attacks. Zinc and **copper** metabolism are related to one another. Reports that supplemental zinc has a beneficial effect on common cold symptoms need to be confirmed.

Where found
Meat, seafood, dairy products, cereals, and whole grains. Supplements are available as **zinc citrate, zinc gluconate,** or zinc sulfate.

Recommended dosage
Recommended daily allowances (mg): adult males 11 and older and in pregnancy: 15; adult females 11 and older: 12;

children 1 to 10: 10; children under 1: 5; nursing mothers: first six months: 19; second six months: 16.

Side effects and overdosage
Zinc toxicity can cause nausea, vomiting, and diarrhea. Too much zinc may cause a **copper** deficiency.

Zinc acetate

OOO

Use
Astringent.

Where found
Benadryl external anti-itch product line (with **diphenhydramine**), Caladryl Clear. Also found in some deodorants and antiperspirants.

Recommended dosage
By itself may be applied as often as needed in a 0.1 to 2 percent solution for adults and children over 2. For combination products, follow manufacturer's recommendations.

Side effects and overdosage
Generally well tolerated.

Zinc citrate

OOO

Use
Inhibits formation of tartar (calculus) on teeth by interfering with calcification of plaque. Also used orally as a nutritional zinc supplement.

Where found

In tartar control toothpastes such as Aim Anti Tartar Formula, Close-Up Anti-Plaque, Close-Up Tartar Control, and Mentadent Tartar Control.

Recommended dosage

Follow manufacturer's recommendations.

Side effects and overdosage

Generally well tolerated.

Synonyms

Zinc citrate trihydrate.

Zinc oxide

ooo

Use

Skin protectant and sunscreen. Also has mild astringent and antiseptic effects.

Where found

By itself or in combination with **petrolatum** and **cornstarch** in zinc oxide paste. Present in many external skin care products such as hemorrhoid and diaper rash preparations. Calamine lotion is a suspension of zinc oxide and ferrous oxide (which makes it pink).

Recommended dosage

By itself, may be applied as often as needed. For combination products, follow manufacturer's recommendations.

Side effects and overdosage

Tends to be safe and well tolerated. If it comes in contact with certain metallic jewelry it may cause a black discoloration of the skin.

Synonyms

Flowers of zinc, zinc white.

Zinc sulfate

○ ○ ○

Use
Astringent and zinc nutritional supplement.

Where found
20/20 Drops, Clear Eyes ACR, Eye-Sed, VasoClear A, Visine Allergy Relief, Zincfrin in combination with decongestants such as **naphazoline, tetrahydrozoline,** or **phenylephrine.** Also found in vitamin and mineral products.

Recommended dosage
Follow manufacturer's recommendations.

Side effects and overdosage
Well tolerated when used as directed.

GLOSSARY

Acute. Starting suddenly, getting worse quickly, or having a short course. Contrast with chronic.

Adsorption. A process in which molecules stick to the surface of another substance. It is distinct from absorption, in which molecules are taken into and incorporated within another substance. **Activated charcoal** and **attapulgite**, for example *adsorb*, whereas **cornstarch** and **talc** *absorb*.

Acidosis. A condition in which acidic ions (charged particles) accumulate in the blood or in which basic ions are lost from the blood. It may be respiratory, in which carbon dioxide is abnormally retained, or metabolic, in which too much acid is produced (as in severe diabetes) or too much base is excreted (as in severe diarrhea) or not enough acid is excreted (as in severe kidney disease). It may also be produced by overuse of the diuretic **ammonium chloride.**

Alkalosis. A condition in which basic (alkaline) ions accumulate in the blood or in which acidic ions are lost from the blood. It may be respiratory, in which hyperventilation causes excessive carbon dioxide excretion, or metabolic, in which either large amounts of acidic ions are lost (as in severe vomiting) or large amounts of basic ions are ingested (as in taking too much antacid).

Analgesic. Something that alleviates pain.

Anemia. Reduced hemoglobin (the iron containing substance responsible for carrying oxygen) in the blood.

Antibiotic. A substance designed to kill bacteria. There is no effect on infections caused by viruses, fungi, or yeasts.

Antihistamine. A substance that antagonizes the effects of histamine. There are two main types. The H_1 types, commonly called antihistamines, block allergic symptoms, whereas the H_2 types, called histamine$_2$ receptor antagonists, inhibit stomach acid production.

Antipyretic. Something that reduces fever.

Antiseptic. A substance designed to kill many different types of microorganisms (germs), such as bacteria, viruses, fungi, and yeasts.

Astringent. A substance causing contraction and shrinkage of tissues, such as on mucous membranes. There is little if any effect on skin that is intact, so that the common use of an astringent as a general aid to good skin care is questionable. Astringents also act by causing precipitates with protein, so that oozing discharges tend to dry up.

Bacteria. Single-celled microorganisms (germs) widely found in water, soil, and other living creatures. Although certainly capable of causing disease, they are mostly an essential element in the balance of nature. Unlike viruses, bacteria do not need other cells in which to live.

Callus. A thickening of the top (horny) layer of the skin produced by friction or pressure. Calluses may occur anywhere and are usually not painful. The medical term for a callus is callosity. Contrast with corn and wart.

Chronic. Lasting a long time or recurring. Contrast with acute.

Corn. A usually painful thickening of the top (horny) layer of the skin produced by friction or pressure. They are almost exclusively located on the feet. The growth is shaped like a cone, with the tip pointed down. Corns are caused by wearing tight shoes, having bony protruberances, or losing the fat pads on the soles of the feet. The medical term for a corn is clavus. Contrast with callus and wart.

Cream. A substance containing water and oil, with water predominating. Creams, as opposed to ointments, tend to dry the skin.

Dermatitis. A general and nonspecific term meaning inflammation of the skin.

Demulcent. Something that soothes. Specifically, it usually refers to a substance that coats and protects mucous membranes, such as the mouth, anus, and parts of the genitals. Examples include glycerin, sugar syrup, liquorice, and honey.

Dyspepsia. Upset stomach. It can refer to nausea, abdominal pain, cramping, heartburn, constipation, diarrhea, gas, and vomiting, alone or in combination.

Electrolyte. A substance that exists as an ion (charged particle) in the blood. Electrolytes mainly include sodium, chloride, potassium, and carbon dioxide (CO_2). Electrolytes have a number of important functions, including that of stabilizing the pH of the blood. Loss of electrolytes can cause severe illness in those with diarrhea or vomiting.

Fungus. A type of plant, including mushrooms, molds, yeasts, and a variety of other organisms, such as those that cause ringworm, athlete's foot, and jock itch. Fungi are larger than bacteria and are usually antagonistic to them.

Histamine. A powerful chemical found in the body that affects the bronchial tubes, blood vessels, digestive tract, and brain.

Humectant. A substance that helps retain moisture. Examples are glycerin and sorbitol.

Infection. A disease that results from invasion by a microorganism (germ), such as bacterium, fungus, or virus.

Infestation. A disease that results from a parasite living on or in the body, such as lice or tapeworms.

Inflammation. A change in tissue characterized by heat, swelling, pain, redness, and decreased function. On the skin, itching is often present also. Inflammation may be due to an infection, but not necessarily.

Impetigo. An infection of the skin caused by bacteria, most often *Staphylococcus* or *Streptococcus*. The hallmark is a superficial crust the color of honey.

Influenza. A severe respiratory disease caused by a virus. It is characterized by sudden (acute) onset, high fever, headache, severe aches and pains, and marked weakness.

NSAID. Abbreviation of the term non-steroidal anti-inflammatory drug. The steroid refers to compounds such as cortisone or prednisone, which are still the most potent drugs available for relieving inflammation. Their side effects, however, make them undesirable, and the NSAIDs are popular because many of these side effects are not present. Although **aspirin** is technically an NSAID (but **acetaminophen** is not) the term is usually reserved for other drugs, of which **ibuprofen, ketoprofen,** and **naproxen** are available OTC. There are many more NSAIDs that are available by prescription and some of these may also change their status in time. Here is a list of those available:

Carprofen (Rimadyl)
Diclofenac (Voltaren)
Diflunisal (Dolobid)
Fenoprofen (Nalfon)
Floctafenine (Idarac)
Flurbiprofen (Ansaid)
Indomethacin (Indocin)
Ketorolac (Toradol)
Meclofenamate (Meclomen)
Mefenamic acid (Ponstel)
Piroxicam (Feldene)
Sulindac (Clinoril)
Suprofen (Suprol)
Tiaprofenic acid (Surgam)
Tolmetin (Tolectin)
Zomepirac (Zomax).

Ointment. A substance that consists of oil and water, with oil predominating. Ointments, in contrast to creams, tend to reduce skin dryness.

Plaque. A film that covers the teeth in which bacteria live.

Protectant. A substance that forms a coating on the surface of skin or mucous membranes to prevent rubbing, chafing, or other irritation by clothing, irritating compounds, or other skin surfaces. Examples include **petrolatum** and **hard fat**.

Tartar. Crusted plaque on teeth that has become calcified. Also called calculus.

Virus. A microorganism, composed of DNA or RNA, that needs to live within a living cell in order to reproduce. Viruses are much smaller than bacteria and can cause a wide variety of diseases in animals and plants.

Vitamin. A substance essential to nutrition in minute amounts.

Wart. A thickening of the top (horny) layer of the skin produced by an infection with a virus. Warts may occur anywhere on the skin or mucous membranes. If on the sole of the foot they are called plantar warts, which, if on weight-bearing sites, may be painful. The medical term for a wart is verruca. Contrast with callus and corn.

Yeast. A type of fungus. The ones responsible for causing disease, such as *Candida albicans,* often exist normally in or on the body and only become a problem when tissues or body chemistry is altered in some way.

APPENDIXES

I THE INTELLIGENT CONSUMER

Every time you take a drug, OTC or prescription, you are performing a unique scientific experiment, one that has never before been conducted in the history of the universe. This is because you are a unique individual, with a unique DNA structure. Because you share most of that structure with other humans, it is expected that you will react like other humans, and for the most part this is true. If you take an internal analgesic for your headache, you should expect your headache to go away. If you take an antacid, you should expect heartburn relief. And if you apply an athlete's foot medication, you should expect to get rid of your athlete's foot fungus. Most of the time you'll be better off, but not always.

It is possible, for example, to activate a latent stomach ulcer with the analgesic, to cause constipation or diarrhea with the antacid, or to develop an allergic skin reaction to the athlete's foot medicine. If your body reacts in this way you'll have lost some ground in your quest for comfort. And it is comfort that you're after when you purchase an OTC preparation.

None of the OTC drugs and ingredients discussed in this book, with the notable exception of **insulin,** will save your life. They can, however, make life a bit more tolerable by alleviating the aches and pains, sniffles, intestinal malfunctions, sleepless nights, or other minor annoyances that can add to the stress and strain of daily existence. So the first step in being an intelligent consumer of OTC drugs is to keep everything in perspective. The second step is to learn as much as possible.

There is no such thing as knowing too much, as long as the information is accurate. Being able to tell fact from fiction—or fraud—becomes the fundamental issue. Unfortunately, a lot of the information most readily available today is misinformation; the sale of popular medical books and magazines is often inversely proportional to their accuracy. If you have a health problem you will have to search for accuracy, and you have to understand that you might not like what you'll find out.

Now, if you could keep a clear head at all times you would no doubt make the right decision about whether to take a particular medicine, but illness gets in the way of things. When we get sick we regress and become dependent on those around us. We look for a quick fix. We become much more suggestible, much more likely to listen to grandma's opinions on our skin rash, the health food store clerk's recommendation for our lack of energy, or the TV commercial's offer on a new fat-absorbing elixir.

Advertising is probably the main source of confusion in the health field today. Part of this is because of a psychological quirk of human beings, the behavior pattern known as brand name loyalty. Robitussin is so synonymous with cough relief and Tylenol with pain relief and Ex-Lax with constipation relief that the active ingredients in these products could change tomorrow and sales would continue as if nothing had happened. Drug companies produce a myriad of drugs and drug combinations under the same product name, which they refer to as a complete product line. Actually, companies do this to provide themselves with a complete bottom line. The different products aren't necessarily bad, just confusing.

There is no such thing as truth in advertising, because advertising is a form of legal lying—you're only getting one side of the picture. A favorite trick of many commercials is to provide testimonials, statements by those who attest that they were cured, relieved, or restored by a particular nostrum. These may be actual people or they may be paid actors. They may be sane or they may be delusional. What testimonials never do is provide a balance: you will not find anyone who says they got ripped off, developed a bad rash, died because they delayed medical treatment, or ended up in the hospital from a drug interaction. As a general rule you should never believe a testimonial and never buy a product based on a testimonial. If you give a hundred bald men distilled water to rub on their heads and tell them it's a newly discovered formula from Sweden to grow hair, about twenty-five of them, on average, will swear it worked. These people become the raw material for testimonials. And with a few dollars for their trouble they'll say just about anything.

It seems that there are people who will believe just about anything and people who will doubt just about anything, but there is a little bit of the believer and disbeliever in all of us. We all would *like* to believe that it's possible to lose eighty pounds painlessly by chewing gum containing chromium three times a day, just as we would all like to believe that it's possible to live forever.

So how does one arrive at the truth? The only way—and it's far from perfect—is through the scientific study, otherwise known as the scientific experiment. Another way to think of a good study is by using the word evidence, and to think of the process as a trial, which it is. Properly controlled and designed clinical trials are difficult and expensive. There are many variables, of which investigator bias (manufacturers pay for many studies) is only one. It is well known, for instance, that many subjects sign up for studies to earn money but don't actually take the drugs because of the possibility of side effects.

There is another type of evidence found in medical literature, and this is the case report. A doctor will report on a case or group of cases in which he or she has observed a certain phenomenon. It may be that a drug, treatment, or operation worked in a particular disease, or it may be that unforeseen problems arose.

But even when a good study has been performed or a seemingly accurate case has been reported, there is the matter of interpretation. Anyone who has watched a trial knows that there are always two ways of looking at evidence, and it's not only the public that has a problem. When is the last time you heard of a unanimous Supreme Court verdict? Almost without exception the justices look at and consider the exact same evidence and come to diametrically different opinions about it.

The only attitude to have about any health claim is clearly to be skeptical. You will hear advocates for a particular point of view saying that studies show this or that, but if you live long enough you'll hear the studies first say one thing, then the opposite, then back to the first thing, then perhaps vacillating somewhere in the middle. A couple of years ago two prestigious medical journals, the *Journal of the American Medical Association* and the *New England Journal of Medicine,* published studies at about the same time about the relationship between estrogen and breast cancer. Each came to a different conclusion.

Always remember two things about studies. First, there is no perfect study. Second, studies don't and can't establish the truth, but rather a kind of general statistical probability. A certain study may show that a certain antibiotic gets rid of a strep throat ninety percent of the time. All this means to you, if you have a strep throat, is that the odds are about nine out of ten that you'll get better if you take that antibiotic.

II THE FOOD AND DRUG ADMINISTRATION

The FDA is the governmental body that decides, among many other things, whether a drug can be sold directly to consumers and how it must be labelled. Although the FDA is concerned with both safety and effectiveness, safety issues are more important to it. Its responsibilities have changed over the years as both laws and the commissioner have changed.

The issues with which the FDA deals are complicated because some substances may be classified as drugs, some as cosmetics, and some as foods or dietary supplements. Manufacturers often go to great lengths to keep their products in certain classifications for economic reasons. For example, because DHEA, melatonin, herbs, and some vitamin and mineral products are listed as a dietary supplements, the rules are different for them than they would be if they were listed as drugs or medications. Consequently, the FDA has less control over their sale, advertising, labelling, and distribution, because the 1994 Dietary Supplement Health and Education Act exempted dietary supplements from strict FDA control and oversight. Before this law was passed, the FDA could require that a manufacturer prove, at its own expense, that a product was safe. Now, the FDA must prove, at our (the taxpayers') expense, that it *isn't* safe.

Laws are usually passed in response to some catastrophe. We legislate with the 20/20 vision of hindsight. The FDA was formed in 1906 to combat adulterated food and quack doctors. The Food, Drug and Cosmetic Act of 1938 allowed it to oversee drugs, and was passed after the deaths of more than a hundred children who had received a tainted sulfa drug. In 1962, after thousands of deformed babies had been born because their mothers had taken thalidomide for morning sickness, the power of the FDA was enhanced.

The whole question of how much governmental regulation we need is open to debate, and there are those who think the powers of the FDA are far in excess of what society needs. But the fact is, the average person is in no position to make an informed decision about drugs. Indeed, even scientists have trouble interpretating complex and sometimes contradictory data.

Another argument against the FDA is that it is too slow in approving potentially life saving medications. The FDA, because it is a human institution, is far from perfect. But as long as a main principle of law and common sense is caveat emptor—let the buyer beware—it is far better to have a strong FDA than a weak one.

We need not go into a long discussion of the drug approval process except to say that, in order for a drug to be considered safe and effective for distribution, its manufacturer must present evidence to the FDA. The FDA then studies the matter and issues its ruling, placing the item in one of three categories. Unlike prescription drugs, OTC drugs themselves aren't evaluated, just their ingredients. The following are the three categories:

Category I products are considered safe and effective.

Category II drugs are not safe and effective.

Category III drugs are in limbo; there are not enough data to make a decision.

Although all approved drugs fall into Category I, this does not mean that they are all equally safe, nor are they all equally effective. **Aspirin** and **acetaminophen** are both in Category I, but **acetaminophen** is far safer, in general, particularly in those who have a history of stomach ulcers. And although both **pseudoephedrine** (for congestion) and **guaiafenesin** (to liquefy sputum) are also Category I, the **pseudoephedrine** is far more effective for its indication than the **guaiafenesin** is for its.

Another helpful service of the FDA is to rate drugs according to safety during pregnancy and breast feeding. This is the classification system used (italics added):

Class A: Adequate *human* studies have been performed and there is no evidence of risk to the fetus.

Class B: Adequate *animal* studies have been performed and there is no evidence of risk to the fetus; if animal studies have shown a risk, adequate human studies have been performed and there is no evidence of risk.

Class C: Adequate *animal* studies have either not been performed or have shown a risk, but adequate *human* studies have not been performed.

Class D: There is evidence of *human* fetal risk but the benefits of the drug may outweigh the risk.

Class X: There is evidence of *human* fetal risk and the risk clearly outweighs the benefit.

This is more than a little confusing. Since adequate human studies have so rarely been performed with many medications and drugs, it is far safer to avoid *all* drugs in pregnancy unless your doctor tells you otherwise.

You can contact the FDA by telephone if you have questions:

General Consumer Inquiries: 301-443-3170
Freedom of Information Act: 301-443-6310
Office of Public Affairs: 301-443-1130

The FDA also maintains a World Wide Web page (http://www.fda.gov/) for those with access to the Internet. This site is extensive and can furnish you with anything you need to know.

III HOW TO READ A LABEL

The FDA has recently proposed a new system of labelling for OTC drugs that will make it easier to read and understand the dose, indications, and side effects of OTC drugs. Manufacturers will gradually be going over to this system or a variant of it. This is an example of the FDA's proposal, but it may change, since it is currently being reviewed.

Active ingredient (in each tablet)   Purpose
Chlorpheniramine Maleate 4 mg   Antihistamine

Uses: for the temporary relief of these symptoms of hay fever
▶ sneezing ▶ runny nose ▶ itchy, watery eyes

Warnings
Ask a doctor before use
if you have:
▲ glaucoma
▲ a breathing problem such as emphysema or chronic bronchitis
▲ difficulty in urination due to enlargement of the prostate gland
If you are:
▲ taking sedatives or tranquilizers

When using this product:
- ▲ marked drowsiness may occur
- ▲ alcohol, sedatives, and tranquilizers may increase the drowsiness effect
- ▲ avoid alcoholic beverages
- ▲ use caution when driving a motor vehicle or operating machinery
- ▲ excitability may occur, especially in children

If pregnant or breast feeding, ask a health professional before use.
Keep out of reach of children. In case of overdose, get medical help right away.

Directions:

Adults and children over 12 years:	Take 1 tablet every 4 to 6 hours as needed. Do not take more than 6 tablets in 24 hours.
Children 6 to under 12 years:	Take ½ tablet every 4 to 6 hours as needed. Do not take more than 3 tablets in 24 hours.
Children under 6 years:	Ask a doctor.

Source: U.S. Food and Drug Administration

IV POISON CONTROL CENTERS

The great majority of the centers listed below are certified by the American Association of Poison Control Centers, which requires twenty-four-hour staffing, a medical director, and nurses and pharmacists available to answer questions.

ALABAMA
Children's Hospital of Alabama
1600 7th Avenue South
Birmingham, AL 35233-1711
205-933-4050
800-292-6678 (Alabama only)
205-939-9245 (Fax)

Alabama Poison Center
408-A Paul Bryant Drive East
Tuscaloosa, AL 35401
205-345-0600
800-462-0800 (Alabama only)
205-759-7994 (Fax)

ALASKA
Anchorage Poison Control Center
Providence Hospital Pharmacy
PO Box 196604
Anchorage, AK 99519
907-261-3193
800-478-3193
907-261-3645 (Fax)

ARIZONA
Samaritan Regional Poison Center
Good Samaritan Medical Center
1111 E. McDowell Road
Phoenix, AZ 85006
602-253-3334
602-256-7579 (Fax)

Arizona Poison and Drug Information Center
University of Arizona Health Sciences Center
1501 N. Cambell Avenue
Tucson, AZ 85724
520-626-6016 (Tucson)
800-362-0101 (Arizona only)
520-626-2720 (Fax)

CALIFORNIA
Central California Regional Poison Control Center
Valley Children's Hospital
3151 N. Millbrook
Fresno, CA 93703
209-445-1222
800-346-5922 (Central California only)
209-241-6050 (Fax)

Los Angeles Regional Drug and Poison
Information Center
Los Angeles County/University of Southern
California Medical Center
1200 N. State Street
Los Angeles, CA 90033
213-222-3212
800-777-6476
213-226-4194 (Fax)

San Diego Regional Poison Center
UCSD Medical Center
200 W. Arbor Drive
San Diego, CA 92103
619-543-6000
800-876-4766 (619 area code only)
619-692-1867 (Fax)

San Francisco Bay Area Poison Control Center
San Francisco General Hospital
1001 Potrero Avenue
San Francisco, CA 94110
800-523-2222
415-821-8513 (Fax)

University of California Davis Regional Poison
Control Center
2315 Stockton Boulevard
Sacramento, CA 95817
916-734-3692
800-342-9293 (northern California only)
916-734-7796 (Fax)

COLORADO
Rocky Mountain Poison and Drug Center
8802 E. 9th Avenue
Denver, CO 80220
303-629-1123
303-739-1119 (Fax)

CONNECTICUT
Connecticut Poison Control Center
University of Connecticut Health Center
263 Farmington Ave.
Farmington, CT 06032
800-343-2722 (Connecticut only)
203-679-1623 (Fax)

DISTRICT OF COLUMBIA
National Capital Poison Center
George Washington University Hospital
3201 New Mexico Avenue, NW
Washington, DC 20016
202-625-3333
202-362-8536 (TTY for the deaf)
202-362-8377 (Fax)

FLORIDA
Florida Poison Information Center
Tampa General Hospital
P.O. BOX 1289
Tampa, FL 33601
813-253-4444 (Tampa only)
800-282-3171 (Florida only)
813-253-4443 (Fax)

GEORGIA
Georgia Poison Control Center
Grady Memorial Hospital
Box 26066
80 Butler Street SE
Atlanta, GA 30335
404-616-9000
800-282-5846 (Georgia only)
404-616-6657 (Fax)

HAWAII
Hawaii Poison Center
Kapiolani Women's and Children's Medical Center
1319 Punahou Street
Honolulu, HI 96826
808-941-4411

INDIANA
Indiana Poison Center
Methodist Hospital of Indiana
P.O. Box 1367
1701 N. Senate Boulevard
Indianapolis, IN 46206
317-929-2323
800-382-9097 (Indiana only)
317-929-2337 (Fax)

IOWA
Poison Control Center
University of Iowa
200 Hawkins Dr.
Iowa City, IA 52242
800-272-6477 (Iowa only)

KENTUCKY
Kentucky Regional Poison Center
Kosair Children's Hospital
Medical Towers South
PO Box 35070
Louisville, KY 40232
502-629-7275
800-722-5725 (Kentucky only)
502-629-7277 (Fax)

LOUISIANA
Louisiana Drug and Poison Information Center
Northeast Louisiana University School of Pharmacy
Monroe, LA 71209
800-256-9822 (Louisiana only)
318-342-1744 (Fax)

MAINE
Maine Poison Center
Maine Medical Center
22 Bramhill St.
Portland, ME 04102
800-442-6305 (Maine only)
207-871-6226 (Fax)

MARYLAND
Maryland Poison Center
20 N. Pine Street
Baltimore, MD 21201
410-706-7701
800-492-2414 (Maryland only)
410-706-7184 (Fax)

MASSACHUSETTS
Massachusetts Poison Control Center
300 Longwood Avenue
Boston, MA 02115
617-232-2120
800-682-9211
617-738-0032 (Fax)

MICHIGAN
Poison Control Center
Children's Hospital of Michigan
3901 Beaubien Boulevard
Detroit, MI 48201
313-745-5711
313-745-5493 (Fax)

Blodgett Regional Poison Center
Blodgett Memorial Medical Center
1840 Wealthy St. SE
Grand Rapids, MI 49506
800-764-7661 (Michigan only)
616-774-7204 (Fax)

MINNESOTA
Hennipin Regional Poison Control Center
Hennipin County Medical Center
701 Park Avenue
Minneapolis, MN 55415
612-347-3141
612-904-4289 (Fax)

Minnesota Regional Poison Center
St. Paul-Ramsey Medical Center
640 Jackson Street
St. Paul, MN 55101
612-221-2113
612-851-8166 (Fax)

MISSISSIPPI
Mississippi Regional Poison Control Center
University of Mississippi Medical Center
2500 North State St.
Jackson, MS 39216
601-354-7660
601-984-1676 (Fax)

MISSOURI
Poison Control Center
Children's Mercy Hospital
2401 Gillham Road
Kansas City, MO 64108
816-234-3430
816-234-3421 (Fax)

Cardinal Glennon Children's Hospital Regional Poison Control Center
1465 S. Grand Boulevard
St. Louis, MO 63104
314-772-5200
800-366-8888
314-577-5355 (Fax)

MONTANA
Rocky Mountain Regional Poison and Drug Center
645 Banock Street
Denver, CO 80204
303-629-1123
800-525-5042 (Montana only)
303-739-1119 (Fax)

NEBRASKA
Mid-Plains Poison Control Center
8301 Dodge Street
Omaha, NE 68114
402-390-5555 (Omaha)
800-955-9119 (Nebraska and Wyoming only)
404-354-3049 (Fax)

NEW HAMPSHIRE
New Hampshire Poison Information Center
Dartmouth-Hitchcock Medical Center
1 Medical Center Dr.
Lebanon, NH 03756
603-650-5000 (ask for the Poison Center)
800-562-8236 (New Hampshire only)
603-650-8986 (Fax)

NEW JERSEY
New Jersey Poison Information and Education System
201 Lyons Avenue
Newark, NJ 07112
800-962-1253
201-705-8098 (Fax)

NEW MEXICO
New Mexico Poison and Drug Information Center
University of New Mexico
Albuquerque, NM 87131
505-843-2551
800-432-6866 (New Mexico only)
505-277-5892 (Fax)

NEW YORK
Finger Lakes Regional Poison Control Center
University of Rochester Medical Center
601 Elmwood Avenue
Rochester, NY 14642
716-275-3232
800-333-0542 (New York only)
716-244-1677 (Fax)

Long Island Regional Poison Control Center
Winthrop University Hospital
259 First Street
Mineola, NY 11501
516-542-2323
516-739-2070 (Fax)

New York City Poison Control Center
455 First Avenue
Room 123
New York, NY 10016
212-340-4494
212-POISONS
212-447-8223 (Fax)

NORTH CAROLINA
Carolinas Poison Center
Box 32861
Charlotte, NC 28232
704-355-4000
800-848-6946

Western North Carolina Regional Poison Control Center
Memorial Mission Hospital
509 Biltmore Avenue
Asheville, NC 28801
704-255-4490
800-542-4225 (North Carolina only)
704-255-4467 (Fax)

NORTH DAKOTA
North Dakota Poison Information Center
Meritcare Medical Center
720 N. 4th Street
Fargo, ND 58122
701-234-5575
800-732-2200 (North Dakota only)
701-234-5090 (Fax)

OHIO
Central Ohio Poison Center
Columbus Children's Hospital
700 Children's Drive
Columbus, OH 43205
614-228-1323
800-682-7625
614-221-2672 (Fax)

Regional Poison Control System
Cincinnati Drug and Poison Information Center
Box 670144
Cincinnati, OH 45267
513-558-5111
800-872-5111 (Ohio only)
513-558-5301 (Fax)

Greater Cleveland Poison Control Center
11100 Euclid Ave.
Cleveland, OH 44106
216-231-4455
216-844-3242 (Fax)

OKLAHOMA
Oklahoma Poison Control Center
University of Oklahoma
940 Northeast 13th Street
Oklahoma City, OK 73104
405-271-5454
800-522-4611 (Oklahoma only)
405-271-1816 (Fax)

OREGON
Oregon Poison Center
Oregon Health Sciences University
3181 Sam Jackson Park Road
Portland, OR 97201
503-494-8968
800-462-7165 (Oregon only)
503-494-4980 (Fax)

PENNSYLVANIA
Regional Poison Control Center
3600 Market Street
Philadelphia, PA 19104
215-386-2100
800-722-7112
215-590-4419 (Fax)

Pittsburgh Poison Center
3705 Fifth Avenue
Pittsburgh, PA 15213
412-681-6669
412-692-7497 (Fax)

Central Pennsylvania Poison Center
University Hospital
Milton South Hershey Medical Center
Hershey, PA 17033
800-521-6110
717-531-6932 (Fax)

RHODE ISLAND
Rhode Island Poison Center
Rhode Island Hospital
593 Eddy Street
Providence, RI 02902
401-444-5727
401-444-8062 (Fax)

SOUTH CAROLINA
Palmetto Poison Center
College of Pharmacy
University of South Carolina
Columbia, SC 29208
803-777-1117
800-922-1117 (South Carolina only)
803-777-6127 (Fax)

SOUTH DAKOTA
McKennan Hospital Poison Center
800 E. 21st Street
Sioux Falls, SD 57117
605-322-3894
800-843-0505 (Iowa, Minnesota, Nebraska, and North Dakota only)
800-952-0123 (South Dakota only)
605-322-8378 (Fax)

TENNESSEE
Southern Poison Center
847 Monroe Avenue
Memphis, TN 38163
901-528-6048
800-288-9999 (Tennessee only)
901-448-5419 (Fax)

Middle Tennessee Poison Center
501 Oxford House
1161 21st Avenue South
Nashville, TN 37232
615-936-2034
800-288-9999 (Tennessee only)
615-936-2046 (Fax)

TEXAS
North Texas Poison Center
Parkland Memorial Hospital
P.O. Box 35926
Dallas, TX 75235
800-POISON1 (800-764-7661)
214-590-5008 (Fax)

Texas State Poison Center
The University of Texas Medical Branch
Galveston, TX 77555
409-765-1420
800-764-7661 (Texas only)
409-772-3917 (Fax)

UTAH
Utah Poison Control Center
5410 Chipeta Way, Suite 230
Salt Lake City, UT 84108
801-581-2151
800-456 7707 (Utah only)
801-581-4199 (Fax)

VERMONT
Vermont Poison Center
Fletcher Allen Health Care
111 Colchester Avenue
Burlington, VT 15401
802-658-3456
802-656-4802 (Fax)

VIRGINIA
Blue Ridge Poison Center
Box 67
Blue Ridge Hospital
Charlottesville, VA 22901
804-924-5543
800-451-1428
804-971-8657 (Fax)

WASHINGTON
Washington Poison Center
155 NE 100th Street
Seattle, WA 98125
206-526-2121
800-732-6985 (Washington only)
206-526-8490 (Fax)

WEST VIRGINIA
West Virginia Poison Center
West Virginia University Health Sciences Center
3110 MacCorkle Avenue SE
Charleston, WV 25304
304-348-4211
800-642-3625 (West Virginia only)
304-348-9560 (Fax)

WISCONSIN
Poison Control Center
University of Wisconsin
600 Highland Avenue
Madison, WI 53792
608-262-3702
800-815-8855 (Wisconsin only)

WYOMING
See *NEBRASKA*

V SAFE USE OF OVER-THE-COUNTER MEDICATIONS

- Never take an OTC product without being thoroughly familiar with every item listed in the active ingredients. Ask your doctor or pharmacist if anything is unclear.

- If you take any prescription medication, make sure you know about possible OTC drug interactions.

- Always check the label before taking a dose.

- Keep medications out of the reach of children in a dry, safe area. Do not keep them in your purse.

- If you're pregnant or nursing, check with your doctor before using any medication.

- Pay attention to expiration dates and throw out anything that has expired.

- Keep medications in the bottles they came in.

- Use child-proof bottles.

- Follow your doctor's or the manufacturer's recommendations carefully.

- Keep ipecac on hand.

- Post the number of your nearest Poison Control Center on every phone.

VI OTC INGREDIENTS THAT MAY CAUSE REACTIONS TO SUNLIGHT (PHOTOSENSITIVITY)

Benzocaine

Benzoyl peroxide

Brompheniramine

Chlorpheniramine

Clemastine

Coal tar

Cyclizine

Dexchlorpheniramine

Dimenhydrinate

Diphenhydramine

Doxylamine

Ibuprofen

Ketoprofen

Meclizine

Naproxen

Phenindamine

Pheniramine

Pyrilamine

Tripelennamine

Triprolidine

Vitamin A

INDEX

411

413

428

435

440

For Ashley, Heather, Laura,
and their (future) progeny

Acknowledgments

I would like first to thank Pam for her comments, suggestions, and support. Thanks also to my medical consultants for their care and consideration; to Drs. Amy David, Steven David, and William Jay Swirsky; to Mitchell Ivers; and of course to Scott and Barbara Siegel. A different kind of thanks go to Barbara, Dan, Pauline, Nicholas, Anastasia, and Michael, and the rest of the gene pool.

THE ![PDR FAMILY GUIDES] PDR

POCKET GUIDE
TO PRESCRIPTION DRUGS™

**REVISED AND UPDATED
WITH THE LATEST NEW DRUGS
THE SAME INFORMATION YOUR DOCTOR RELIES ON**

*Based on Physicians' Desk Reference®,
the Nation's Leading Professional Drug Handbook*

♦ Side effects, drug interactions, dosages—all in everyday English

♦ Quick, easy alphabetical references by familiar brand names—with convenient generic cross-references

♦ Hundreds of actual-size full-color drug photographs

♦ 40 new entries, including protease inhibitors, Redux,™ Allegra,™ and drugs for asthma, acne, and more

Available from Pocket Books

POCKET
B O O K S

1275-02